HERBAL
TEAS

101 Nourishing Blends
for Daily Health and Vitality

Kathleen Brown
Recipe development by Jeanine Pollak

STOREY
BOOKS

The mission of Storey Communications is to serve our customers by publishing practical information that encourages personal independence in harmony with the environment.

Edited by Deborah Balmuth
Cover design, illustration, and production by
    Carol Jessop, Black Trout Design
Text design by Jen Rork
Photographs by Giles Prett except for: photos
    of individual herbalists; pages 3 and 99 by
    John Conte; pages 63 and 108 by A. Blake
    Gardner
Professional assistance by Jeanine Pollak
Indexed by Susan Olason/Indexes &
    Knowledge Maps

The information in this book is true and complete to the best of our knowledge. All recommendations are made without guarantee on the part of the author or Storey Books, Inc. The author and publisher disclaim any liability in connection with the use of this information. For additional information, please contact Storey Books, Inc., Schoolhouse Road, Pownal, Vermont 05261.

This publication is intended to provide educational information for the reader on the covered subject. It is not intended to take the place of personalized medical counseling, diagnosis, and treatment from a trained health professional.

Storey Books are available for special premium and promotional uses and for customized editions. For further information, please call Storey's Custom Publishing Department at 1-800-793-9396.

Printed in Canada by Transcontinental Printing
10 9 8 7 6 5 4 3 2 1

Library of Congress Cataloging-in-Publication Data

Brown, Kathleen L.
        Herbal teas : 101 nourishing blends for daily health & vitality / Kathleen Brown: recipe development by Jeanine Pollak.
                p.   cm.
        Includes bibliographical references and index.
        ISBN 1-58017-099-4 (pbk. : alk. paper)
        1. Herbal teas—therapeutic use.   I. Pollak, Jeanine, 1957–   .   II. Title.
RM666.H33.B765
615'.321—dc21   99-18420
                                                                                                                    CIP

CONTENTS

HERBALIST PROFILES

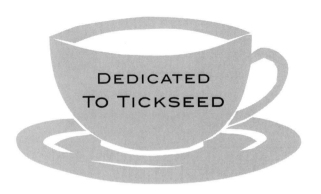

**DEDICATED
TO TICKSEED**

ACKNOWLEDGMENTS

I especially want to honor Jeanine Pollak for her immense contribution to this book, not just for sharing her magnificent collection of recipes, but for the opportunity I had to appreciate and learn from her passion for herbs and joyful approach to life.

Green blessings go to Deborah Balmuth and Robin Catalano of Storey Books for their contributions in making my dream of writing this book come true. Their excellent, and thankfully endless, ideas and kind advice have been such a wellspring of support and encouragement that words are insufficient to express my gratitude.

Something that sets this book apart are the short profiles of herbalists that are woven within the recipes. Some are well known in the green nations, others are just starting on their herbal paths. All are united in their connection to herbs, however, and their histories, accomplishments, and dreams were inspirational to me. I was personally honored by the opportunity to learn about them through working on this book, and their lives touched me, as I know they will touch you. It's a privilege to have them grace these pages with their favorite tea recipes, as it is to them and every other person who passes on what they've learned from the plants that this book is truly dedicated.

Preface

My introduction to herbal tea started many years ago when I was told, for health reasons, to limit my caffeine intake. The biggest problem was "going out for coffee" with friends and dealing with the local coffee shops that had no herbal tea. For years, I had to carry tea bags around in my purse and feel the scorn of waitresses everywhere when I requested only "hot water, please." Sometimes they even made me buy the Lipton tea bag just to get the water!

During those early years, an avid herbalist friend tried to help me with those health problems I was experiencing. He suggested I make therapeutic herbal teas, with strange-sounding ingredients found only in shops on back streets — small dark places full of glass jars and really odd odors, the type of place you'd be likely to find eye of newt! But, it was the beginning of a journey for me, not only my initial foray into the world of herbs but also an awareness of the part I could play in being responsible for my own health. There was no echinacea tea at the local supermarket then, and the process of finding and preparing the herbs to aid digestion, encourage sleep, or ward off a cold was challenging, a real adventure.

I'm actual thankful that I had the health problems I did early in my life. It started me down the path of lifelong learning about herbs and alternative medicine, and most important, forced me to adopt the habit of being responsible for my own health.

Happily, you've probably noticed that herbal tea is more available nowadays. Herbs are also more popular in the mainstream population, on the cover of nearly every magazine in the grocery checkout line and even brand-name over-the-counter remedies sport the word "herbal" on their labels. Fortunately for all of us, but particularly those of you just discovering the benefits of herbal tea who think it has to come in a bag, even fresh and bulk dried herbs are much more easily found, usually in well-lit health food stores on the main roads.

So why this book, when there are already excellent books around on herbal tea? I've collected many books on herbal tea myself and treasure every one. Many of them do have tea recipes, but this book is really *about* recipes, addressing everything from flu and colds to pimples and mood swings! These pearls of wisdom and healing were developed by recipe goddess, Jeanine Pollak, who really believes in having fun with herbs. You can tell that by the names she's given them — A Pimple's Worst Nightmare Tea, or Post-Potluck 911.

The information in Getting to Know the Tea Herbs — a little history, therapeutic benefits, the part used, taste, and specific brewing instructions — comes from the accumulated knowledge of many, in a variety of ways. Books, personal experiences, years of practice, videos, classes, workshops, whole conferences devoted to sharing herbal wisdom, and literally sitting at the feet of those in the know — these are my sources. I've found that herbalists, on the whole, are incredibly generous with their time and knowledge, so it's been a wonderful and rich path to follow, seemingly and thankfully without end.

I personally feel that in drinking the medicine of the plants, you also gain the desire to know more about these green allies. Perhaps it's something that happens in the natural order of things, that in gaining the medicine, you gain an awareness, and a desire is born for continuity, to learn and pass on the knowledge. This is the herbalist tradition. May this book illuminate your path, enriching your spirit and body, and may you enjoy every sip of herbal tea in good health and old age.

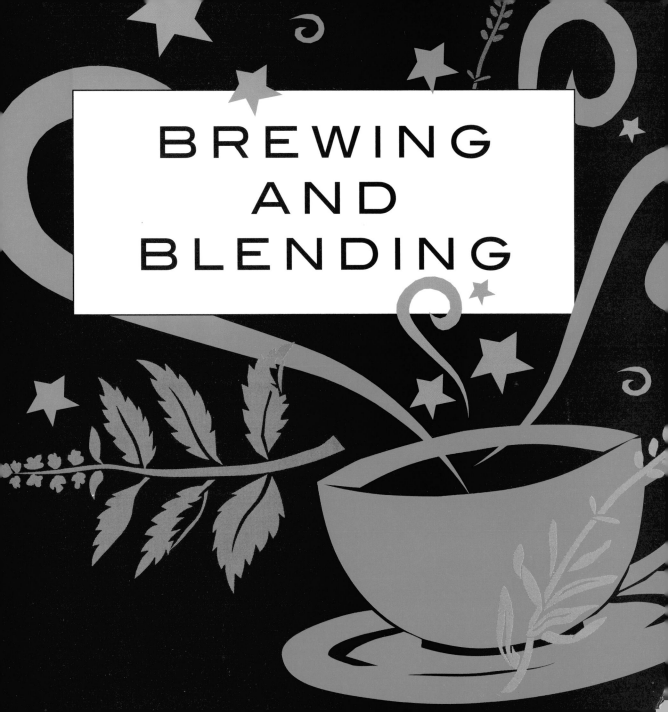

BREWING
AND
BLENDING

There are essentially two ways to prepare the perfect cup of herbal tea: an infusion, *where the herbs are steeped, and a* decoction, *which means the herbs are simmered for a period of time. Both techniques are covered in detail below, along with information on the tools and utensils you'll need, whether to use fresh or dried herbs, the ratios to use, what kind of water is best, and so forth. Let's start.*

INFUSE OR DECOCT?

An infusion is the best technique for brewing teas when leaves, flowers, or crushed berries or seeds are used. These ingredients easily release their essential oils and valuable nutrients while steeping in hot water. The basic rule of thumb is to pour boiling water over the herbs, cover the pot, and allow to steep anywhere from 10 to 30 minutes. The longer a tea steeps, the stronger it will taste, but herbalists agree that, for some formulas, a longer steeping time allows nutrients to be extracted more fully.

Decoctions, on the other hand, are the method of choice when brewing teas from roots, barks, and more woody parts of herbs. In this case, the plant material must be simmered in boiling water to release its valuable properties.

You're probably wondering, what if you're using a combination of ingredients, both leaves and roots, for example? The basic technique is actually to both infuse and decoct — simmer the roots 20 minutes in a covered container, remove the pot from the heat, add the leaves, stir well, cover, and steep 10 to 20 minutes.

This next tip is important so will probably be mentioned more than once: use organic herbs if possible. As herbalist Gail Ulrich explains, your tea is only going to be as good as the herbs you put in it. If you're gathering fresh herbs in the wild, be absolutely certain they have not been sprayed or exposed to pesticides or pollution, such as those growing alongside a road. If you're using roses and some of the other flowering plants and trees, be especially careful they haven't been sprayed.

**Infusion
Rule of Thumb**

Pour boiling water over the herbs. Stir well, cover the pot, and steep 10 to 30 minutes.

Tools of the Trade

Besides a little knowledge, you'll also need some tools and utensils. There are many types of strainers and other tools for brewing tea, some fancy, others very simple. A fine-mesh metal strainer is the tool of choice for many herbalists who believe the herbs need to float happily and unencumbered while brewing, without being confined by the ubiquitous tea ball or spoon. Some like bamboo strainers, others collect brewing gadgets (okay, I confess), but whether your tea tool is aesthetic or practical, simple or ostentatious, it's up to you. Tea balls and spoons are convenient to use at work or when traveling, though some hard-core herbalists have been known to carry a porta-pot, teapot that is!

Another way of taking your tea with you to work or when traveling is to make your own tea bags. You can purchase empty 1-cup-size tea bags, or buy or make small cloth bags with drawstrings into which you put your tea blends. Cheesecloth cut into small squares and fastened with string, thread, or, in a pinch, a rubberband works too. Place 1 teaspoon of tea blend into the bag or fabric, and you'll have tea to go!

Decoction Rule of Thumb

Add the herbs to boiling water, stir well. Cover the pot, and simmer on low heat from 20 to as long as 60 minutes if, for example, you're using large, whole roots such as ginseng.

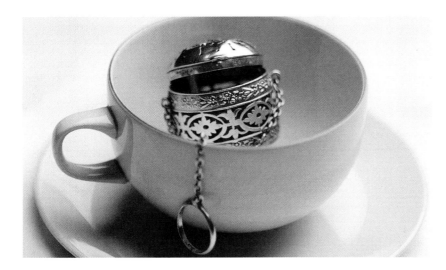

Berries and Seeds

It's best to crush berries and seeds and infuse with the leaves and flowers rather than decoct them with the roots, which destroys the more volatile properties released during crushing.

Choosing the Right Container

I, along with probably every other avid herbal tea drinker in the world, collect teapots and other tea "toys." It's always nice to bring out that special teapot when friends drop by for tea. For me, my teapots have different experiences associated with them, such as gifts from family or friends or purchased on a special adventure. Each has a story or memory associated with it, so when I make tea, I not only enjoy the beneficial beverage, but I reexperience those moments, too.

Glass, stainless steel, enamel, and most pottery (check to make sure the glaze is lead free!) are the best types of containers in which to make tea. Glass is particularly wonderful because you additionally experience the visual aspect of watching the tea brewing and becoming. Rosemary Gladstar says of her teapot collection that her quest is to find the most beautiful that is the most useful. The more useful in its function, the more beautiful the teapot becomes, a fitting vessel to hold the "useful" plants.

You don't need a fancy teapot, however, or any teapot, for that matter. The simple quart canning jar is not only the most utilitarian for brewing tea, it may be the best for preserving the aromatic oils and other volatile properties of the plants as well. It's simple: Just put the herbs in a jar, pour boiling water over, stir well, cover, and steep. As far as how long to let it sit, use the suggestions for standard infusions and decoctions discussed earlier until you become familiar with the tastes and times involved in brewing your favorites.

FRESH OR DRIED HERBS?

Dried herbs will never equal fresh in providing the nutritive value, vitality, flavor, color, and texture, so using fresh herbs in your tea is always preferable. Let's face it, though, there are times and places when fresh herbs just aren't an option. There's a good part of the world where winter descends with a vengeance and decimates all living things for up to half a year or more. Or you may live in an urban jungle of high-rises, surrounded by concrete, not exactly in a position to wildcraft or grow your own herbs. Some herbs are only raised in tropical rain forests or other exotic locales and must be imported in dried form anyway. What then?

If you are lucky enough to have your own garden, you can harvest and dry the bounty yourself, thus assuring organic quality and freshness. (Check the chapter on gathering for basic drying techniques and storage considerations.) Or you might try purchasing locally grown herbs from reputable growers. If these are not options, attempt to obtain the best-quality dried herbs available, organic if possible, again, from reputable sources. There are several mail-order sources included in the Resources section for your reference.

Dried herbs do have the advantage of longer storage time, and it's acceptable to use both fresh and dried together. Always refrigerate leftover teas, for up to 2 to 3 days.

Measuring Systems

As you become more familiar with the art of making tea, the "handful" method most herbalists enjoy as their system of measurement will seem more understandable. Before long, you, too, will be throwing a handful of this or that into the pot and won't even need the proportions that are given in our recipes. For now, though, the ratios provided will help you get more, shall we say, *rewarding* results. To be as consistent as possible and avoid confusion, the ingredients are shown as "parts" rather than precise measurements such as teaspoons, cups, or whatever. This is also for your convenience, so you can make any quantity you desire. For instance, if 1 part valerian, 1 part hops, and 1 part chamomile are listed, it just means that the combination will contain one-third of each herb. If your total amount is 3 tablespoons of herb, then you'll use 1 tablespoon of each herb.

The Sun and the Moon in Your Cup

Besides traditional infusions and decoctions, there are a couple of other methods that are fun and interesting to try. You can infuse your teas by sun and moon power! If you want to add roots, bruise or crush them first.

For sun tea, place all the herbs in a large glass jar, fill with water, cover tightly, then put the jar in direct sunlight. You can leave the tea in the sun for several hours, until it's the way you want it to taste.

The moon adds its own form of lunar energy. While the tastes are more delicate and subtle, lunar infusions are enchanting! Place all the herbs in a jar or beautiful crystal bowl, add water, cover, and leave outside all night where it will receive direct light from the moon. In the morning, enjoy your moon magic. Lunar infusions are best during the full moon.

As Good as It Gets
Use only organic herbs and
plant parts with:

★ No chemical sprays
★ No pesticides
★ No exposure to pollution
  (as alongside a road)

In the fresh versus dried question, the ratio is usually 1 teaspoon dried equals 2 teaspoons fresh (roughly double) per 1 cup of water, or 1 ounce of herb to 1 quart of water. We'll use these as standards, although a recipe can vary with strength, density, taste, and color of the herbs in the mix. This is really a guideline, so adjust accordingly and feel free to experiment.

If making teas for daily tonic purposes, to bolster and nourish the body, drink 2 to 3 cups per day. If you're sick, drink 4 to 6 cups per day, or drink as much as you can. Get a good thermos, and take your tea with you. For children ages 3 years and up, usually ¼ to ½ cup is given. For elderly people, or if the tea is very strong and bitter, ½ cup is recommended. These are general guidelines, however, so note the specific instructions given with each recipe.

H_2O

Since the basis of all teas is water, start with the purest water you can. If you are lucky to have good tap water, use it. If not, consider distilled or bottled water.

If not expressly noted in a recipe's instructions, use 1 quart of water to start with, making the herbal ingredients (parts) equal approximately 1 ounce of plant material.

TO BLEND OR NOT TO BLEND

Here's how it goes. You start drinking herbal tea, for whatever reason. You become more interested, even obsessed, and pretty soon, you're wanting to take it to the next level — blending your own! It's a real possibility, and, as you'll read in the histories of many of our guest herbalists, probably even inevitable that you'll eventually find yourself wanting *to blend*. You might even feel compelled to grow your own herbs, learn all you can about them, eat and drink them, heal yourself with them, heal others with them, write a book about them! Guest herbalist Gail Ulrich says they will change your life. I've found that to be true.

So, here you are, you've turned to this section on blending to get a peek at how difficult it might be. You'll be happy to learn that it's really quite a simple art. You've gained some experience making tea with your green friends and acquiring all the proper tools, so now there's really only two additional things required to start blending your own teas. The first is gaining a bit of knowledge and getting familiar with the herbs. Many herbalists recommend picking a few herbs with which you become really "intimate." As Colorado herbalist Tammi Hartung says, it's better to know many uses for one herb than one use for many herbs.

Getting to Know the Herbs

One of the things that kept me from blending my own teas at first was feeling like I didn't know enough about the properties of each herb. But, you don't have to start with complex medicinal formulas. It's not nearly so intimidating to mix a few herbs together to make a great-tasting beverage that's inviting to the senses. You can still reap the therapeutic benefits behind the scenes, so to speak.

I think one of the best ways to really know your herbs is to grow them in your garden, seeing them in every season, from seed to flowering and everything in between. Your garden might only be some containers on your apartment balcony or a few pots in a windowsill. No matter how modest, it's great to have your plants handy. Get familiar with the aroma of each herb, experience the texture and color, taste it. Besides providing the ingredients for tea-and-food medicine, herb plants add a dimension of simple, fragrant presence. In reading the biographies of the guest herbalists, you'll note that many of them mention they feel the plants themselves were their greatest teachers. The chapter Getting to Know the Tea Herbs (pages 109 to 147) will give you a good introduction to the therapeutic qualities of the herbs used in our recipes. Once you've mastered the basics, you may want to get a more intensive herb guide (some great ones are listed in the Resource Books section) to learn more about possible therapeutic results with particular herbs.

Beyond knowledge and experience, the only other thing that's essential to blending your own teas is to get creative! Allow your mind to run free. As owner of a Connecticut herb shop, Martha Paul says the sky's the limit as far as creating teas — a good attitude to adopt when beginning to blend. The number of possible combinations is practically unlimited.

Ready, Set, Blend!

Here are a few things to consider when starting to blend your own teas. And don't forget, the key word is *experiment*!

★ Get to know your herbs: how they taste, smell, and feel; what blends well and what doesn't. You will find that some flavors completely overpower the more delicate ones.

★ You can start with a goal, for instance, of making a tea to help you get to sleep. Or not. You might just want to make something refreshing for enjoying on the porch in the summer or before the fire in the winter.

★ Use the stronger, primary flavors as the foundation, then add secondary herbs to create unique and interesting flavors, aromas, and textures.

★ Taste will always be your ultimate test.

The chart at right is included to familiarize you with some of the basic tastes and to help you in blending tea herbs. So, for example, if you like lemony, mint teas, you can choose one (or more) herbs from both the Citrus and Minty columns.

TASTE CHARACTERISTICS

SWEET
Anise
Licorice
Rehmannia
Stevia*
Vanilla

MINTY
Catnip
Peppermint
Spearmint
Violet
Wintergreen

WOODY
Crampbark
Echinacea
Ephedra
Gingsengs
Sarsaparilla

ROOTY
Burdock
Dandelion
Dong Quai
Gingsengs
Oregon Grape
Yellow Dock

SPICY
Allspice
Cardamom
Cinnamon
Coriander
Fenugreek
Ginger
Vitex
Yerba Santa

FLOWERS
Chamomile
Elder
Hawthorn
Jasmine
Lavender
Linden
Red Clover
Rose

LICORICE
Anise
Fennel
Licorice
Star Anise

TART
Hibiscus
Rose Hips

CITRUS
Lemon Balm
Lemongrass
Lemon Peel
Lemon Verbena
Orange Peel

GRASSY
Alfalfa
Horsetail
Oatstraw

* Stevia, though not included in our Getting to Know the Herbs section, is an incredibly sweet herb that is often used to sweeten drinks or in cooking. Only a pinch is necessary, and you can usually find it in most health food stores.

Some of the herbs and spices that are used in our recipes are added primarily for flavor, like allspice, cardamom, cinnamon, coriander, star anise, and vanilla, though they may have therapeutic benefits as well. For the recipes that call for citrus, use oranges, lemons, tangelos, mandarin oranges, and so forth interchangeably. Use only organic citrus fruit since most commercial citrus is chemically preserved and you do not want to use that peel.

Beyond Teas

In some of the recipes, you'll find suggestions that tinctures or elixirs may also be made from the same blend of herbs. As Gail Ulrich of Blazing Star Herbal School says, the stronger and less pleasant tasting herbs may best be prepared as tinctures or capsules. There are some excellent books on making medicinal preparations, so we won't go into a lot of detail here, but just include a brief introduction to get you started if you want to make tinctures and the like.

Tinctures

This is tincture making at its most *simple,* which, interestingly, is the term traditionally applied to single-ingredient tinctures, or simples. In a way, a tincture is a tea, only stronger. In a tea, the herb's properties, or values, are extracted in water, with heat. In a tincture, the values are extracted into a different medium, over time.

Tincturing may seem too "serious" for you at first. Making your own medicine is compelling, however, and ultimately very empowering. The act of tincturing may not appeal to you the first (or tenth) time you read this, but someday you may move in that direction and when you are ready to give it a try, you'll know where to find these directions. Information is like a seed, I've always thought, and, once planted, may eventually bear fruit, even if it's years later.

It's incredibly easy. You may find it even easier than making tea. Tincturing has some other important advantages. It's more potent and sometimes more palatable than tea. A bottled tincture is infinitely portable, assimilated immediately, can be preserved almost indefinitely, and is attractively cost-effective.

Caution

Never use isopropyl alcohol for internal use.

Step-by-Step Tincture Making

1. If using fresh herbs, coarsely chop or mince. If using dried herbs, powder them first in a coffee grinder. Either way, you are trying to release the essential oils and volatile goodies.

2. Place processed herbs in a widemouthed jar in which the herbs make up about ¼ of the total volume. For example, if the herbs represent ½ cup, the container should hold 2 cups total. Cover the herbs with two times as much liquid if using fresh herbs and three times as much liquid if using dried herbs. Use the liquid of your choice: apple cider vinegar, glycerin, and alcohol such as vodka or brandy are the most common. Blend well. If tincturing dried herbs with glycerin, dilute ⅔ parts glycerin with ⅓ part water, but use the glycerin full strength if using fresh herbs. If tincturing with alcohol, use at least 80 to 100 proof (40 to 50 percent alcohol), like vodka. Forty percent alcohol is usually sufficient to effectively extract an herb's constituents. When tincturing very resinous herbs such as black sage or yerba santa, or herbs from which it's harder to extract their properties, however, you'll need a higher percentage of alcohol, probably 70 to 90 percent. Brandy has a slightly sweeter taste that many herbalists prefer for throat and lung blends, digestive bitters and some tonic formulas, and, though it is only 80 proof (40 percent alcohol), it is sufficient for most tinctures.

3. Close jar tightly. If you're tincturing in vinegar, you may want to cover the top of the jar with plastic wrap to prevent the corrosive action of vinegar that could rust the lid shut.

4. Shake daily for 2 to 4 weeks, strain, then bottle, preferably in dark glass. Traditionally, the full moon is considered a good time to bottle tinctures. (Don't forget to label your bottles, or you won't know what you've got when you're done!). Store at room temperature. If you prefer, bottle into smaller dark, glass bottles with eye dropper tops for more convenient use.

Tincture Dosages

Obviously when you've got a wide range of human health, weight, and constitutions to factor into an equally varied range of herb properties and strengths, the proper dosage for a tincture will vary just as much. Generally, though, 1 to 2 dropperfuls of tincture one to five times per day is appropriate. You may add the tincture to a little water or tea. Be aware, however, that a dropperful of bitter tincture can make an entire cup of tea bitter. We suggest pouring off 2 tablespoons of tea and adding the tincture to that. Let the tea sit 5 minutes, and most of the alcohol evaporates. Now you're drinking 2 tablespoons with a strong taste, not an entire cup. Or, you can add the tincture to the last few sips of tea. You'll thank us for this tip! This technique also works great for those not wanting to take alcohol.

Flavor-Enhancers for Elixirs

★ Rosehips, fresh or dried

★ Berries, fresh or frozen

★ Orange or tangerine slices, fresh, organic

★ Warming spices such as ginger and cinnamon

★ Fresh summer fruit such as peaches, pears, plums, nectarines

★ Dried fruit (in the winter)

Elixirs and Syrups

Elixirs and cordials are basically the same, and throughout the text, we've used the terms interchangeably. An elixir is a delicious, fruity and festive concoction, typically a tonic formula to nourish and support a particular body system such as heart, brain, or immune system, for example the Heart and Soul Tonic in the Senior Advantage section.

Making an elixir. The basic method is to choose your herbs, cover with three times as much brandy, add any of the yummy and nourishing flavor-enhancing ingredients from the list in the box, and tincture as you would normally, for 2 to 4 weeks. When done, strain, and add 1/10 part maple syrup or honey. Take 1 teaspoon to 1 tablespoon once or twice per day.

The flavor-enhancing supplemental ingredients shown at left should be added as one-half the amount of the herb parts, for example, 1 part echinacea, ½ part ginger, ½ part blackberries. Be aware that some herbs, like valerian or goldenseal, are not good candidates for elixirs, as no amount of flavorful additions can make them more palatable!

Making a syrup. Here's an interesting technique for making syrups, what could be described as the "superbowl of herbal teas." These are the thick and soothing, highly flavorful and potent beverages, usually made with fruit and sipped as needed for tonic benefits.

First, prepare a tea, simmering for 1 to 2 hours in a covered pot. Remove from heat and allow to steep another 1 to 2 hours, stirring occasionally. Strain out all the solids, squeezing all the liquid through cheesecloth. Measure the volume of tea, for instance, 1 cup. Then add ½ to ¾ as much molasses and ¼ part brandy as a preservative. Recipes will vary slightly but this is the basic method.

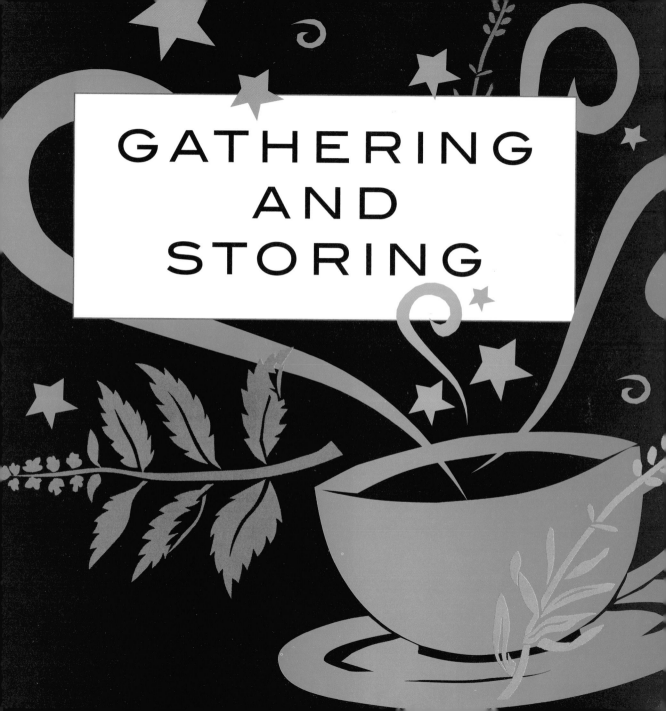

GATHERING AND STORING

Almost all the herbs in our recipes can be grown in your garden for the absolutely freshest ingredients, or they can be fairly easily obtained at your local natural foods store, more frequently fresh, but consistently in dried form. Many of them can also be wildcrafted, that is, found growing in the wild and gathered ethically. As many herbalists caution, though, if wildcrafting: Be absolutely certain what plants you're collecting. Some herbs look identical, but their properties can vary greatly from beneficial to toxic and even deadly poisonous. For your convenience, mail-order sources are also listed in Resources. Whatever source you choose, try to find organic if possible, certainly the best quality available. Your teas will only be as good as the quality of the herbs you're using.

Harvesting Herbs

Pick out your favorite basket or trug, and go out into your garden on a dry, sunny morning. The best time of day is after the dew has evaporated, but before the sun is hot enough to dry all the volatile oils and properties from the plants. This is just a rule of thumb, however, and varies from plant to plant. Gathering from mid-morning to early afternoon is fine for something like mints, for instance, where a little sun and warmth brings the volatile oils to the peak of perfection. Don't pick the herbs when they're wet if you're planning to dry them, since they may become moldy. If you're going to use them fresh, you can pick them even in the rain!

Contrary to what you might think, cutting the leaves and flowers from the herb actually is beneficial to the plant and helps them to grow even more vigorous and abundant. Besides, it improves the morale of plants when yellow and dying leaves are picked off, making room for new, healthy leaves. Your plants will thank you for taking such good care of them!

Think of it as giving the plant a haircut, but a trim, not a full buzz cut! Use scissors when gathering the herbs, to get a clean break, rather than picking with your fingers, which could pull up the roots. And gather the tips rather than full stems to get the most tender parts. If harvesting from small plants, leave at least two sets of leaves at the base of each stem so the plant has something with which to continue growing. You'll be amazed how quickly the plants produce new growth, so that you can harvest several crops from a plant each season. Be especially careful not to pick herbs that have been exposed to weed killers or chemicals of any kind, car exhaust, or excessive dust.

For aromatic, leafy herbs such as mint, the best time to harvest is just before the plant flowers, as this is when the greatest abundance of natural oils is concentrated in the leaves. This is especially important when the herbs are to be dried and stored, as the oils provide the best flavor, therapeutic value, and color.

Using Fresh Herbs

Okay, you've got the herbs in your basket and have tidied up your plants. Now what? If you want to make tea from fresh herbs, first wash them thoroughly in clean cold water, then shake or pat them dry with a towel. Herbs that grow close to the ground like parsley and thyme need to be washed carefully because they are the most likely to have soil on their leaves. Remove stems and any dead and imperfect leaves, chop or bruise the herbs, and pop the green goodies into a teapot. It's that simple. But, if you want to dry and store them, read on.

Drying the Herbs

An important thing to remember when drying herbs is to process them as quickly as possible after picking to ensure maximum flavor. Once gathered, shake gently to remove dust and insects. It's important to keep the herbs out of strong light and sun to prevent the color and flavor from fading. Be sure to keep the herbs separate and well identified, because, as they dry, many look the same.

To Dry Herbs Quickly. Spread on a mesh rack and place in a slow oven set from 100° to 125°F. Using more heat causes the volatile oils in the plants to be destroyed. Leave the oven door open, and stand nearby because some leaves dry quickly.

To Air-Dry Herbs. Make sure the herbs are not left in places that could be attacked by insects or rodents. Vermin are especially common in hot, humid climates. In cold climates, mildew is a factor to consider.

The drying area should be dry, well ventilated, and out of direct light. In damp or cold climates, some artificial heat may be necessary to supplement the natural drying process. If you're hanging the herbs in bunches, don't make your bunches too large, or the leaves could turn black or moldy. You can hang air-drying herbs inside paper bags to keep the dust off, but just be sure to punch many holes into the bags to let the air in and keep moisture out.

Some herbs dry very well when spread on trays, but don't spread them too thickly. Parsley leaves, for instance, are so thick they can be spread only one layer deep. Thyme, however, holds so little moisture you can just leave a big pile to dry in a basket.

When drying small-leaved herbs such as thyme, pick branches instead of leaves and hang them in bundles to dry. Once they're dry, it's easy to strip the leaves from the stems by running your fingers gently backward down either side. The larger-leaved herbs like mint and sage are better picked separately from the branches before drying. In a warm, dry spot, most herbs will air-dry in anywhere from 4 to 7 days, depending on climate. Heavy-leaved herbs may take several weeks, however. To check if your herbs are totally dry, crumble a bit between your fingers. If they're crispy and break cleanly, they're dry. If they bend and are still flexible, they need more time to dry. Leaves, properly stored, may last 1 to 2 years but are usually best used within 1 year. If you're drying your own herbs, at least you know the date they were dried. When buying dried herbs commercially, you really don't know when they were processed.

Lunar Tip

Leaves gathered when the moon is waning tend to dry most rapidly since they retain less sap in their leaves and stems.

Flowers

Harvest flowers when they are fragrant and most lovely. If they're past their prime, they won't be as aromatic and flavorful. Shake gently to remove any dust or insects. Long-stemmed flowers such as lavender dry best hung upside down in bunches. Rose petals and other flowers with more delicate blossoms are best dried on screens and in baskets. Remember, don't dry in direct sun. A dry, shady place with good air circulation is best. Recipe goddess Jeanine recommends putting flower petals in a ventilated brown paper bag and drying them in the back seat of your car! Be sure they are well dried before storing. Flowers are best when used within one year.

Seeds

Gather seeds when they're barely ripe, as soon as they begin to look brownish, because just a day or so later, they will be blowing all over, and it'll be too late. Instead of preserving your harvest, you'll have planted next year's army of new plants! Pick seeds early in the morning, snipping off the entire seed head. Drop them into a paper bag or cut the whole plant and place it, upside down, in a bag. Puncture the bag and hang it in a warm, airy, shady place. Once dried, all the seeds fall to the bottom of the bag. Seeds can remain viable for years, since they have natural wrappings to hold in their oils.

Roots

A plant from which roots are to be gathered usually needs to reach a certain maturity before its valuable properties are developed, several years in some cases. Autumn is usually the best time to harvest roots, once you've determined that the plant is sufficiently aged. Dig or gently pull up the plant, shake off any excess dirt, then cut off part of the root, leaving enough to support the plant's continued growth. Then replant. Wash the roots in cool water, trimming off side roots,

Freezing Herbs

Freezing works very well for some herbs — dill, lemon balm, lemon verbena, mint, rosemary, and thyme to name a few. Wash the herbs well, and pat them dry with towels. You can freeze them whole or chopped. Plastic bags work well, as they take up little space when stacked flat. Or add a little water and freeze the herbs into ice cube trays. When frozen, pop the cubes from the trays into plastic bags, and take a few out when needed. Another good technique for freeze storing is to put about 1 part chopped herb in 2 parts butter and freeze. The butter preserves the color and flavor and is great for cooking, too.

which don't have much flavor. Split the roots in half lengthwise and chop so they'll dry more quickly. To preserve flavor, keep them in coarsely chopped pieces until you're ready to use. At that time, powder them in a coffee grinder to release the flavor. Properly stored in dark glass jars a dark, cool place, roots can last 2 to 3 years.

STORING

Here are some simple, but very important considerations in storing dried herbs.

★ The type of container is vital, with glass or metal being the best. Dark glass is especially good, since it prevents light from fading the herbs' vitality. If using clear glass, store in a dark place, if possible, but at least, out of direct light.

★ Herbs must be completely dry or they will mold.

★ Store immediately after drying to best preserve volatile oils, color, texture, and flavor.

★ Use airtight containers to keep dust and vermin out.

★ Package each herb separately and label every container carefully.

★ Store in a cool, dry, dark place for best results.

★ Monitor containers regularly to make sure there is no condensation.

Lunar Tip

Try to gather roots when the moon is waxing, since the roots are the most tender then.

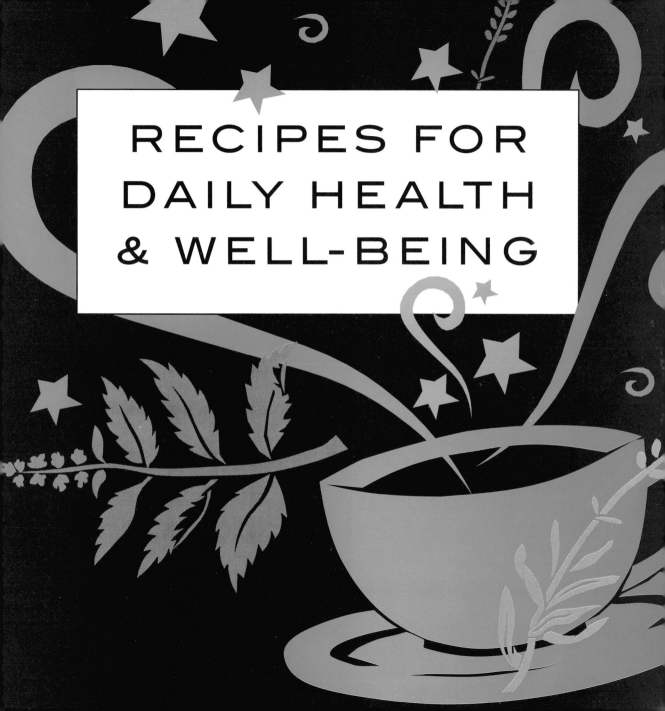

RECIPES FOR DAILY HEALTH & WELL-BEING

*A*nyone who enjoys a good cup of herbal tea has probably recognized the unique opportunity staring at them from their cup. Herbal teas can be enjoyed for pure pleasure, and they can do you a service at the same time. Even the simple act of taking the time to brew, then sip a cup of tea each day is therapeutic in itself. Slow the day's pace, sip a beverage that is good for your body, mind, and spirit, and you may begin to look at things in a different way.

GIVE US THIS DAY OUR DAILY BLENDS . . .

The teas in this section are as nourishing as they are tasty and simple to prepare, making it easy to incorporate this pleasant and healthy habit into your daily routine.

NOURISHING DAILY BLEND

1 **part burdock root**

1 **part chamomile flowers**

1 **part nettle leaves**

1 **part oatstraw**

1 **part red clover blossoms**

1/10 **part cinnamon chips (optional)**

This recipe tastes great with cinnamon added, but if you are drinking it daily, only add the cinnamon occasionally, as it's too strong and drying for daily use.

1 Add the burdock root to boiling water, reduce heat, and simmer for 15 to 20 minutes in a covered pot.

2 Turn off the heat and add the rest of the herbs.

3 Stir well, cover, and steep 15 to 20 minutes more.

VIOLET-ROSE VITALITY BOOSTER

A superior, vitamin-rich booster for daily health enhancement, this blend is absolutely delightful!

1. Combine all herbs in a pot, and pour boiling water over.

2. Stir well, cover, and steep 15 to 20 minutes.

1 part oatstraw

1 part rose hips (organic)

1 part violet leaves and flowers

¼ part orange slices (organic)

⅛ part rose petals (organic)

SMOOTH SAILING OVER THE DAILY GRIND

Delicious either hot or iced, this tea is a simple way for you to take charge of your daily health and well-being. Both taste buds and nerves will thank you!

1. Combine all herbs in a pot, and pour boiling water over.

2. Stir well, cover, and steep 15 to 20 minutes.

1 part lemongrass leaves

1 part lemon verbena leaves

1 part oatstraw

1 part red clover blossoms

⅛ part spearmint leaves

ALL THIS IN A CUP OF TEA
Rosemary Gladstar
Barre, Vermont

While these few short paragraphs couldn't possibly capture the milestones in her career, much less the essence of Rosemary Gladstar, let it suffice to say that she was the person most named by other guest herbalists as their inspiration and muse. Her biography reads like an herbal time line, beginning with a childhood spent outdoors on her parents' farm and an early love of plant life. The major impetus that

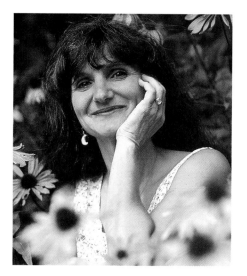

launched her herbal career was a dream to travel by horseback on the Pacific Crest Trail from California all the way to Canada. She got a job as a cleaning lady at a natural foods store to save money for her trip and, because of her familiarity with plants and herbs, she was quickly promoted to "store herb lady." She eventually opened her own herb store, Rosemary's Garden, in 1972. She modestly attributes that success as "a simple dream with a life of its own."

Rosemary is compelled by the plants. Not only is her first name an herb, but she has brown eyes with green centers and admits to wondering if this represents plants growing out of dirt. She describes herself as myopic in her view of the world. "Most of what I see when I look into the world is the green nations," she says. "I think I was born so the plants could use me. I'm really their servant, here to do their bidding."

Rosemary says she was basically a shy introverted person with a passion for herbs, although anyone who's had the privilege to see her in action would question this. "I was asked to come out and share my passion with others. It changed my life forever."

And who, you might wonder, are the mentor's mentors? Rosemary credits her grandmother, Mary Egitkanoff, and Juliette de Bairacli Levy, confessing that she wrote Juliette a "love letter" over 20 years ago. They've been correspondents and friends ever since.

Rosemary thinks teas are the basis of all herbal medicine, citing that water itself is a universal substance that is one of the most healing elements. She further believes that tea involves all the elements: fire, water, earth, and air. "Herbal tea involves the user," she adds. "One has to assume responsibility when one makes tea."

"Tea is warming to the soul and is reflective of all that lives and grows around it," Rosemary explains. "When I drink my tea, I am one with the seasons, the sea by which the herbs grew, the sun and moon under which it was nourished. All this in a cup of tea."

GOOD MORNING BLEND

Rosemary recommends this refreshing and lightly energizing blend to enhance any morning.

⬤ Infuse and steep 15 to 20 minutes.

3 parts peppermint leaves

3 parts rose hips (organic)

½ part freshly grated ginger root

½ part ginkgo leaves

¼ part rosemary leaves

⅛ part orange peel (organic)

a few star anise pods

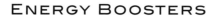

Energy Boosters

Need a little energy? How about early in the morning, to get the day started right? Or for that midafternoon slump at work when the clock says it's been 2:30 for the past hour? Need a little something to keep you going when you're driving a thousand miles straight through? These blends will add some much-needed energy to your endeavors, whatever they might be. You'll also get the added benefit from herbal alternatives in that they'll support you while providing the zip, which commercial stimulants don't provide!

Stamina City

- 1 **part dandelion root**
- 1 **part sarsaparilla root**
- 1 **part Siberian ginseng root**
- ½ **part cooked rehmannia root**
- ⅛ **part cinnamon chips**
- ⅛ **part licorice root**

This hearty blend tastes great and is excellent for general energy as well as being very fortifying for the adrenals, blood, and metabolism. You overworked, stressed-out types, this is for you!

❶ Add this blend to boiling water, reduce heat, and simmer for at least 30 minutes, covered, over low heat.

❷ Remove from the heat, and steep 30 minutes.

Damiana Daytime Delight

While damiana has had a long-standing reputation as an aphrodisiac, it is actually a very good nerve-strengthening herb. When used properly, damiana gently tones nerves and increases overall circulation and sense of well-being.

2 parts oatstraw

1 part damiana leaves

1 part gotu kola leaves

1 part lemon balm leaves

1 part red clover blossoms

1 Combine all herbs in a pot, and cover with boiling water.

2 Stir well, cover, and steep 15 to 20 minutes.

Sassy Root Revival

A strong, root-y tooty, flavorful, hearty blend that nourishes the liver, adrenals, and blood. It's a particularly great tea for the autumn and winter months.

1 part sarsaparilla root

1 part Siberian ginseng root

1 part Korean Red or Chinese Red ginseng root

1 part yellow dock root

¼ part ginger root, freshly grated

⅛ cinnamon chips

⅛ part licorice root

⅛ part orange slices (organic)

1 Add everything but the orange slices to boiling water, reduce heat, and simmer at least 1 hour, covered, over low heat.

2 Remove from the heat, add the orange slices, and steep 10 to 15 minutes.

Tammi Hartung
Canon City, Colorado

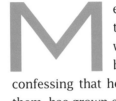

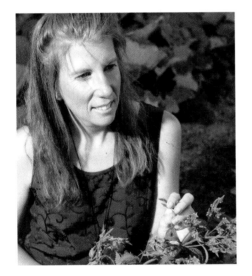

Medical herbalist, teacher, and consultant Tammi Hartung dates her early interest in herbs to the first grade, when she exhibited a project containing 40 species of botanical specimens. She still has that very herbarium, confessing that her fascination with plants, both using and growing them, has grown stronger with each passing day. "Being an herbalist is definitely a life's work," says Tammi. "It's a contagious, terminal, and totally enchanting process." She especially credits her Great-Aunt Ruth for first introducing her to the magic of herbs, offering the past 19 years spent pursuing her herbal passions as homage to that early guidance.

Tammi joined forces with husband Chris, who managed Denver's Chatfield Arboretum for many years, to establish Desert Canon Herb Farm in Canon City, Colorado, combining their considerable plant wisdom. "After so many years of playing with herbs, I feel blessed to be able to earn a livelihood doing my passion," she says. Her credentials include formulating a line of 300 products for an herbal extract company and authoring a series of herbal leaflets, which are published in the United Kingdom. Tammi, an inspirational teacher, also offers apprenticeship programs and an extensive class schedule through her herbal school. She describes how wonderful it is to see her knowledge positively affect the health and well-being of the people she works with, saying "If you're blessed to be given the gift of plant knowledge, then it's your responsibility to share that knowledge with others in a positive, ethical way. I hope my work is always a reflection of the voices of plants in the green nation."

While she is pleased to see five thousand years of documented herbal use gaining more recognition and acceptance throughout the world today, Tammi also feels concern about the environmental impact this popularity will have on wild spaces and the plants that live there. "I do think our culture must be careful in our fast-paced approach to using herbs so that we don't neglect to honor the traditions of herbalism."

Her advice to the beginning herbalist is to learn a small core group of herbs that you use often. "Learn 40 uses for 1 herb rather than 1 use for 40 herbs," she says. Staples in Tammi's pharmacopoeia include nettles for their tonic and nutritive qualities, oatstraw for the nervous system, and other oft-used favorites such as red clover, lemon balm, mint, and ginger.

Tammi believes teas are a delicious, effective avenue for supplying the body with nutrients and medical constituents. "The process of taking tea is soothing and ritualistic," she adds.

TAMMI'S TOTAL TONIC

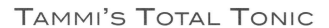

Tammi's philosophy about steeping: Allow a much longer steeping time for therapeutic teas. This provides better mineral extraction to improve the health-enhancing benefits.

1 part oatstraw
1 part red clover blossoms
1 part nettle leaves
½ part mint leaves

❶ Brew ½ cup herb mixture per 2 quarts boiling water. Pour water over herbs and cap jar tightly. Allow to steep a minimum of 4 hours and up to 12 hours.

❷ Strain and drink at room temperature, cool, or rewarmed. Sweeten with honey or maple syrup, if desired.

STRESS BUSTERS

I wonder at what point the concept of "stress" became such an insidious part of all of our lives. You can hardly turn anywhere — TV, radio, print — without being reminded of just how much of the "s-word" we all deal with on a daily basis. There's work, family, money, traffic, hail, earthquakes, day runners, the news, friends, cell phones, health, travel, diet, coffee, body image, pimples, and lest we forget, e-mail. To combat this barrage, we present Stress Busters, some flavorful solutions for the worst of times (and the best of times, too). These blends are delightful any time for any reason. They're useful, and they're gonna help.

SOOTHING WAYS

1 **part catnip leaves**

1 **part lemon balm leaves**

1 **part linden blossoms**

1 **part oatstraw**

1 **part passiflora leaves**

1 **part St.-John's-wort flowers**

A delightful and gentle blend for relaxing the nerves, this tea can be used during the day or before bed to help ensure a good night's rest.

1 Combine all herbs in a pot, and cover with boiling water.

2 Stir well, cover, and steep 15 to 20 minutes.

CALMING CHAMOMILE DELIGHT

This soothing and nourishing formula feeds nerves and has the wonderful refreshing apple taste of chamomile. Good for the day-light hours or pre-bedtime use.

1 Combine all herbs in a pot, and cover with boiling water.

2 Stir well, cover, and steep 15 to 20 minutes.

1 part chamomile flowers

1 part oatstraw

1 part red clover blossoms

1 part skullcap leaves

½ part spearmint leaves

½ part violet leaves and flowers

⅛ part rose petals (organic)

SUPREME SOOTHING NERVINE BLEND

Drink this mineral-rich blend often to support the heart and blood, liver, and nerves.

1 Decoct dandelion root first for 30 minutes, simmering over low heat.

2 Remove from the heat, add the other herbs.

3 Stir well, cover, and steep 10 to 15 minutes.

1 part dandelion root and leaves

1 part hawthorn leaves, flowers, and berries

1 part horsetail

1 part linden blossoms

1 part nettle leaves

1 part oatstraw

1 part red clover blossoms

MERRY MELLOW DAYS

1 part kava-kava root

1 part lemon balm leaves

1 part oatstraw

1 part passiflora leaves

1 part valerian leaves and root

½ part yerba buena, apple mint, or spearmint leaves

If you can use fresh valerian leaves and root and fresh yerba buena leaves, it works better for this particular formula. Since kava is a strong herb, it's best to use this blend only occasionally, maybe a few times a month.

❶ Combine all herbs in a pot, and cover with boiling water.

❷ Stir well, cover, and steep 15 to 20 minutes.

LANGUID LEMON STRESS-AWAY TEA

1 part lemon balm leaves

1 part lemongrass leaves

1 part lemon verbena leaves

1 part oatstraw

1 part passiflora leaves

1 part rose hips (organic)

1 part skullcap leaves

⅛ part orange peel (organic)

This tea is delicious iced or hot and can be enjoyed daily. It's wonderfully nourishing and supportive, toning and strengthening the whole nervous system.

❶ Combine all herbs in a pot, and cover with boiling water.

❷ Stir well, cover, and steep 15 to 20 minutes. Steeping the rose hips preserves the vitamin C better than decocting does.

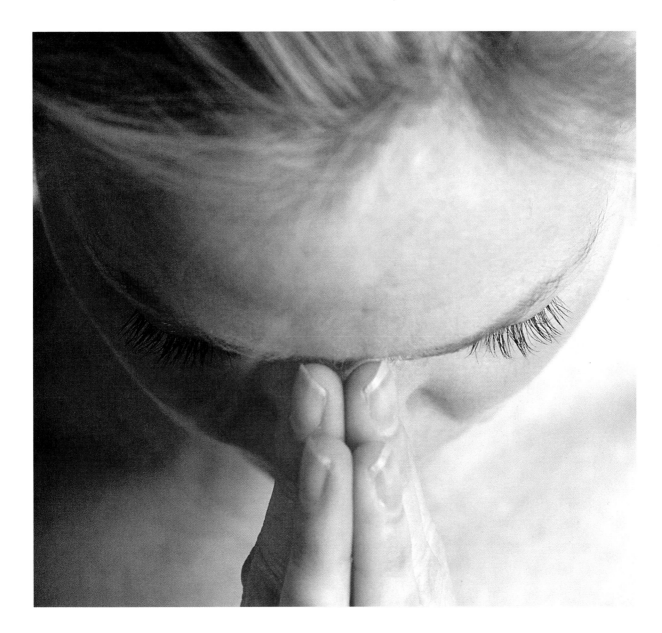

Pam Montgomery
Pawlet, Vermont

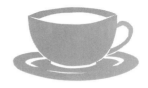

Pam Montgomery, who has most recently established the Partner Earth Education Center, has been involved with herbs for more than 25 years in a variety of ways, including her role as plant spirit medicine practitioner.

She teaches herbal workshops, apprenticeship programs, and classes and is a popular speaker at conferences all over the world. "I love turning people on to herbs," she says. "I'm continually awed

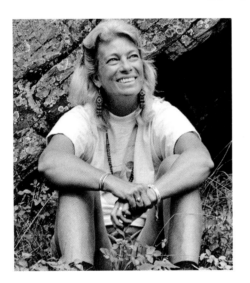

and excited by herbs, and this is why I teach." She relates an interesting experience while teaching a geared-up botany class called Flower Erotica at the Women's Herbal Conference. Upon observing the flowers' sexual parts with a magnifying lens, students gasped, oohed, and aahed in surprise at the exquisite beauty. "It sounded like a garden full of women having orgasms," Pam laughs.

Pam is perhaps most well known for creating an herbal business called Green Terrestrial in 1987, which included tea blends, tinctures, and a set of Moon Flower Essences infused by the light of the moon. Though she recently sold this enterprise, she remains their consultant. Author of *Partner Earth: A Spiritual Ecology,* Pam has three additional book projects in the works.

In 1989, Pam created the annual Green Nations Gathering, was president of the North East Herbal Association in 1993, and two years later joined the board of directors for United Plant Savers.

"Plants have been my doorway to spirit," Pam says. "They are so much more than chemical constituents that have a physical effect on the body." She explains that working with herbs in a co-creative partnership can affect physical, emotional, mental, and spiritual aspects of one's life.

"I particularly like herbal teas because they are supportive in a nourishing way," she says. "I like to incorporate them on a food level so that they become a part of everyday life." Pam relates a special tea she created called Auntie Lyme for those dealing with the challenges of Lyme disease, both boosting energy and reducing joint pain.

Among her favorite herbs, Pam lists nettle as the best all-around nourisher, oatstraw because it's soothing to the nerves, red clover as a good blood cleanser and liver herb, and violet because it's "yummy" and rich in vitamins A and C. Her advice to the beginning herbalist: "Don't be afraid to experiment and don't get caught up in what the 'experts' say." She recommends using good-quality herbs, preferably those you've harvested yourself. "It makes a difference," she adds.

HAPPY DAYS TEA

Pam explains that this tea was created for Green Terrestrial many years ago and says, when the weight of the world is upon you, this tea helps brighten your attitude.

● Blend all herbs in a pot and cover with boiling water. Stir well, cover, and steep 15 to 20 minutes.

1 part borage leaves
1 part calendula blossoms
1 part nettle leaves
1 part oatstraw
1 part basil leaves

Sweet Dreams

We all have nights when we can't sleep, whether it be from stress, illness, or just running through the scenarios of asking the boss for a raise the next day. There's nothing worse than "trying" to get to sleep. You can count as many sheep as you want, practice body relaxation techniques, or read your computer manual, but those eyes continue to remain agonizingly wide open! So here are a few creative blends to take care of the situation. How about a tea called Simple Bliss? You want some, don't you? I know I'd give it a try. Even the ritual of making a cup of tea before bedtime is relaxing, a chance to wrap up the day and affirm a good night's sleep so you'll be ready for whatever tomorrow may bring.

Kava Oasis Slumber Tea

2 parts kava-kava root

2 parts chamomile flowers

1 part lemon verbena leaves

1 part oatstraw

1 part passiflora leaves

1 part rose hips (organic)

½ part spearmint leaves

This is a wonderfully relaxing, sleep-inducing blend to help you unwind. Kava is famous for inducing vivid, colorful dreams, and it really works! It's also good for getting the most of your sleep, even if doze-time is only a few hours. Remember, kava is best used only occasionally, perhaps a few times a month. If you leave out the kava, however, you can drink this tea daily.

❶ Combine all the herbs in a pot, and cover with boiling water.

❷ Stir well, cover, and steep 15 to 20 minutes.

Simple Bliss

Sip this tea slowly, and feel the relaxation seep through your body. It's a fantastic, delicious variation on herb tea, very soothing and safe for daily use.

1 Pour boiling water over the chamomile, cover, and steep 15 to 20 minutes, until strong.

2 Add the soy milk and sweetener.

1 part chamomile flowers

¼ cup vanilla soy milk, cream, milk, or half-and-half per cup

Honey or maple syrup, to sweeten

Nighty Night

This blend is both relaxing and nourishing to the nerves and heart. The Chinese believe that the heart is the home of the "shen," or spirit, and that insomnia is caused by the "restless wanderings of the shen." By nourishing the heart, the shen is more likely to find its desired place of rest.

1 Combine all the herbs in a pot, and cover with boiling water.

2 Stir well, cover, and steep 15 to 20 minutes.

2 parts valerian root

2 parts kava-kava root

1 part chamomile flowers

1 part hawthorn leaves, flowers, and berries

1 part lemon verbena leaves

1 part red clover blossoms

1 part violet leaves and flowers

½ part spearmint leaves

THE SKY'S THE LIMIT
Martha Gummersall Paul
Pomfret, Connecticut

"The sky's the limit as far as creating teas," Martha Paul states convincingly. "I love herbal teas because they are so versatile, and you can drink what your body needs." She describes the process of preparing and drinking tea as relaxing, thought-provoking, and even mesmerizing.

She thinks she was an herbalist in a past life. She grew up in her grandparents' home-style restaurant and became familiar with herbs at an early age, then 11 years ago established Martha's Herbary. Husband Richard became involved in the shop, too, and Martha realized her dream of a workplace where she could raise her daughter, Saga, who's already developing an interest in herbs.

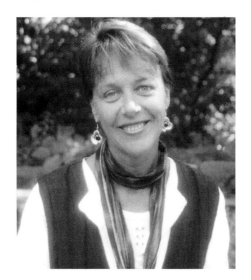

Martha's Herbary is an herbal oasis of charming gardens and a delightful shop filled with garden goodies. You will, most likely, be greeted at the door by Martha's infectious smile and unbounded enthusiasm. She teaches more than 120 classes per year and an eight-month herb garden apprenticeship program, puts out a newsletter, manages her seven-days-a week store, and is a popular speaker across the country. She also has written a cookbook, with volume two in the works. Martha says that seeing her dream of the herb shop become reality and seeing her work "in print" are two treasured milestones on her herbal path. "It's a journey each new day, with something to learn, experiment with, or taste," she says, sharing her passion for herbs and the challenge she feels to keep learning. Visit Martha on her Website at http://www.marthasherbary.com.

Martha visualizes the thrilling sight of wild tansy growing in Nova Scotia and teasel out of control in Pennsylvania as inspiring her early interest in herbs. She also cites the late Adelma Simmons as inspiration. "I admired her accomplishments and her kingdom," Martha states. The Herb Society of America has also been influential in her love and study of herbs.

Martha shares this end-of-season ritual, which she calls Final Tea from the Garden. "I go into the garden with a favorite basket and pick a little of this and a little of that," she says. She then coarsely chops the leaves and stems and adds some edible flowers, dries the mixture on a screen, and stores it in a big jar. Then, during the winter, sitting by the fire, she drinks the tea from this mixture, remembering her garden and the gathering ritual. She claims that students, friends, and family rave about this tea, which is a little different each year.

MARTHA'S MAJOR MELLOW

Martha cautions that this will make you sleepy, so don't plan on going anywhere or doing anything after drinking it!

- Put between 1 teaspoon and 1 tablespoon herb blend for each cup of tea in a ceramic teapot. Pour boiling water over and steep, covered, 15 minutes.

2 parts lemon balm leaves

1 part oatstraw

1 part chamomile flowers

1 part skullcap leaves

½ part valerian root

½ part hops flowers

Oh My Aching . . .

Okay, weekend warriors, you've overdone it. Again. The bicycle ride turned out to be more "up" than "down" and you never realized how small that seat really is! You just survived the Thanksgiving touch-football game on the front lawn but are seriously suffering for your efforts. Whatever. Help! You're hurting. We've got some stuff in this section that works from the inside out and vice versa. Jeanine says the idea for the name of her Spaz-Away products "just came to her" one day. Usually, she explained, the product comes first, then the name, but in this case, it was the name first. Known in her region for creating delicious products with fun names, she says her Spaz-Away theme comes from the fact that the formulas are all anti-spasmodic in nature, whether it be spasms of the body, mind, or emotions. We recommend you sit in a hot Spaz-Away bath, sip a cup of tea, and let go of all that nasty tension. Then dry off with a big fluffy towel.

Spaz-Away Tea

1 part chamomile flowers
1 part kava-kava root
1 part lemongrass leaves
1 part oatstraw
½ part spearmint leaves

This is an excellent tea for relieving the tension of aching muscles. For muscle strain, add 1 part valerian root.

❶ Combine all herbs in a pot, and cover with boiling water.

❷ Stir well, cover, and steep 15 to 20 minutes.

RETURN OF SPAZ-AWAY TEA

Whether it's your muscles or your nerves (I'm sure they're related) that are spazzing-out, this gentle blend soothes and relaxes.

1 Combine all herbs in a pot, and cover with boiling water.

2 Stir well, cover, and steep 15 to 20 minutes.

1 **part chamomile flowers**

1 **part passiflora leaves**

1 **part St.-John's-wort flowers**

1 **part valerian root**

COUSIN OF SPAZ-AWAY

You're going to experience some serious muscle relaxation with this blend, so be prepared to unwind! Adding a bit of honey helps make the taste of the hops more palatable.

1 Combine all herbs in a pot, and cover with boiling water.

2 Stir well, cover, and steep 15 to 20 minutes.

1 **part catnip leaves**

1 **part chamomile flowers**

½ **part hops flowers**

½ **part red clover blossoms**

½ **part spearmint leaves**

⅛ **part lavender flowers (organic)**

1/10 **part orange slices (organic)**

The Terrible Tummy . . . Digestive Woes Addressed

How about after the potluck where you always try a little of everything? Forget the sheer quantity and variety and all you've learned about food groups that don't go together. A total mishmash, let's face it. I mean, really, three kinds of desserts? On top of four different appetizers, three salads, two casseroles, and a grain dish that looked a lot like tabbouleh? And were there mushrooms in that one casserole? You know you always get tummy troubles from mushrooms. This is when you go to the special place where you keep this book, turn to this section, and crank up the teapot. If my tummy was suffering from the potluck blues, I know I'd be comforted by Post-Potluck 911. Why don't you give it a try?

Tummy Tune-Up

1 part catnip leaves

1 part fennel (fresh leaves, stalks, flowers, and seeds, or dried seeds)

1 part ginger root, freshly grated

1 part peppermint leaves

¼ part orange slices (organic)

A great general digestive aid, this tea tastes good too!

1 Combine all herbs in a pot, and cover with boiling water.

2 Stir well, cover, and steep 15 to 20 minutes.

SOOTHING TUMMY TEA SUPREME

This tea is soothing to the digestive tract, both stimulating and assisting digestion.

1. Add the first four ingredients to boiling water, reduce heat, and simmer for 5 minutes in a covered pot.

2. Turn off the heat, add the spearmint, and steep, covered, 15 to 20 minutes.

1 part fennel (fresh leaves, stalks, flowers, and seeds, or dried seed)

1 part fenugreek seeds

1 part flax seeds

1 part ginger root, freshly grated

½ part spearmint leaves

POST-POTLUCK 911

What happens when four carminatives get together? They have a rollicking good time making sense out of all those weird food combinations you just ingested at the potluck dinner!

1. Add the first three ingredients to boiling water, reduce heat, and simmer for 5 minutes in a covered pot.

2. Turn off the heat, add the spearmint, and steep, covered, 15 to 20 minutes.

1 part anise seeds

1 part fennel (fresh leaves, stalks, flowers, and seeds, or dried seeds)

1 part ginger root, freshly grated

1 part spearmint leaves

Yummy Tummy-Tamer Tea

1 part rose hips (organic)

1 part spearmint leaves

½ part star anise

⅛ part licorice root

⅛ part orange slices (organic)

This really yummy, very effective tea for indigestion and stomach-ache is safe to drink daily.

❶ Combine all herbs in a pot, and cover with boiling water.

❷ Stir well, cover, and steep 15 to 20 minutes.

After-Dinner Digestive Delight

1 part spearmint leaves

⅛ part licorice root

A simple, delicious, and very flavorful digestion-enhancing tea! Spearmint is oh-so-soothing, and licorice adds both a sweet flavor and anti-inflammatory properties.

❶ Combine the herbs in a pot, and cover with boiling water.

❷ Stir well, cover, and steep 15 to 20 minutes.

Jeanine's Belly Blast

The blend of herbs in the Better Bitters recipe makes a great tincture in brandy. Simply blend the herbs in the proportions given, and put into three times as much brandy in a widemouthed jar. Shake daily for two to four weeks, then strain through cheesecloth, squeezing out the excess liquid. Rebottle. Take ½ teaspoon in a little water once or twice a day.

BETTER BITTERS FOR THE TUMMY BLUES

Specific for sluggish digestion, this tea will help stimulate digestive enzymes. Because it is a strong formula, small amounts will suffice. Try ½ cup twice a day, about 20 minutes before meals.

1 Add the first three ingredients to boiling water, reduce heat, and simmer for 15 minutes in a covered pot.

2 Turn off the heat, and add the remaining ingredients.

3 Steep, covered, 15 to 20 minutes.

1 part angelica root

1 part ginger root, freshly grated

1 part yellow dock root

½ part fennel (fresh leaves, stalks, flowers, and seeds, or dried seeds)

⅛ part orange slices (organic)

1/10 part cinnamon chips

1/10 part cardamom pods

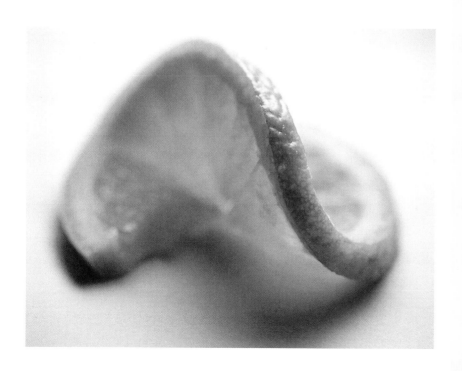

THE GREEK TRADITION
Christa Sinadinos
Arcata, California

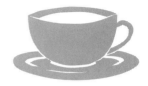

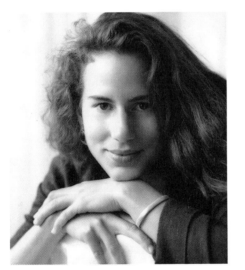

I t was her Greek grandmother who first sparked the interest in herbs that has led to Christa Sinadinos' 10-year involvement. "My grandmother preserved the Greek tradition and passed on her wisdom of herbs and foods," Christa says. "She incorporated herbs as an integral part of her life, praying and blessing all her food." Christa explains that her grandmother is now 86 years old, still radiant and beautiful, and still tending a small herb and vegetable garden.

"I honor and deeply admire her for the way of life she taught me," she adds. Christa also credits Michael Moore for the "volumes of information" and inspiration he shared when she attended his school, especially for showing her "the way herbs dance in our bodies."

Splitting her time between massage therapy and herbalism, Christa works part-time in a local herb store. "I feel fortunate to live in a community that supports my work," she says. "I believe people should do what they love as their work." Explaining that she is passionate about herbs, Christa says that she "created her vocation by following her heart."

Christa enjoys teaching classes about herbs, both locally and nationally at the Women's Herb Symposium. "Teaching allows me to share the tools people can use to heal themselves," she says. She believes most people want to heal themselves and are well capable of doing so with the assistance of their plant friends. Christa feels with the small amount of preventive medicine available in Western medicine that it's inevitable people will turn to herbs. "Herbs and nutrition offer valuable support in building strength and maintaining optimum health," she explains. "If the information is available to them, people can take charge of their health."

A prolific creator of recipes in her own right, Christa believes that herbal teas are a delightful way to ingest herbs, deeply nourishing and soothing. "The ritual of making and drinking tea offers a daily opportunity to nourish oneself," she continues. Christa maintains a full herbal pharmacopoeia in her practice, citing marshmallow, ginger, astragalus, nettles, oatstraw, and chamomile among her favorites. For the beginning herbalist, she offers this advice: "Try each herb individually before trying to blend them."

CHRISTA'S DIGESTIVE DELIGHT

She recommends using fresh ginger in this tea, which is great for any tummy trouble.

- Make a strong decoction by combining all ingredients in a pot, cover with water, and simmer over low heat for at least 20 minutes.

1 part fennel seeds

1 part anise seeds

1 part cinnamon chips

1 part orange peel (organic)

1 part licorice root

3 tablespoons fresh or dried ginger

Fightin' Off the Cold & Flu Brews

Let's face it, even those in the best of health get a cold once in awhile. There is nothing worse than the sniffling-sneezing-coughing-sore throat-aches-and-can't-sleep stuff of a good ol' cold. I honestly believe that when your head's full of, well, you know, you don't think as clearly. These teas will make the body you're captive in feel a little better. Okay, so the Steamin' Mama's Lemonade is not really a tea, but guaranteed to unclog what you thought was terminal. As for Ginger-Angelica Cold Slayer, well, the name says it all, don't you think?

CYCLONE CIDER DELUXE

1 part ginger root, freshly grated

1 part onion, freshly chopped

1 part fresh rosemary leaves

1 part fresh sage leaves, chopped

½ part grated horseradish

2-4 orange and lemon slices (organic)

2-4 cloves of garlic

2-4 freshly chopped cayenne peppers

This is an exotic blend guaranteed to ward off colds, flu, and probably even vampires! Dilute 1 to 2 tablespoons in 1 cup hot water, and sip slowly as needed. You can also add it to salad dressings and marinades for a spicy and exotic taste. Add 1 to 2 tablespoons to soup for an extra boost when you're sick, and it will provide a "hot and sour" flavor.

1 Cover all ingredients with apple cider vinegar in a wide-mouthed jar.

2 Shake daily two to four weeks, then strain, squeezing out all the excess liquid.

3 Rebottle.

4 Add honey to taste, if desired.

ANTIVIRAL ONSET TEA

A takeoff on an old traditional herbal recipe, this tea is for those times when you feel the cold or flu just getting ready to lay siege to your bod. It's warming, diaphoretic, and antiviral.

1 part elder flowers

1 part ginger root, freshly grated

1 part peppermint leaves

½ part yarrow flowers

① Combine all herbs in a pot, and cover with boiling water.

② Stir well, cover, and steep 15 to 20 minutes.

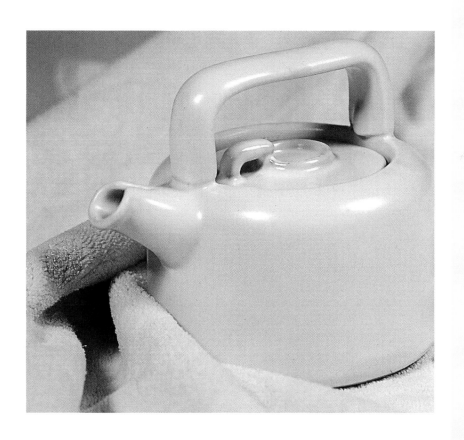

GINGER-ANGELICA COLD SLAYER

1 **part angelica root**

1 **part ginger root,
freshly grated**

1 **part rose hips (organic)**

½ **part fennel (fresh leaves,
stalks, flowers, and seeds,
or dried seeds) or anise
(seeds)**

⅛ **part licorice root**

⅛ **part orange slices (organic)**

If you were a measly ol' virus bug, I bet you'd flee for your life in the presence of this fiery formula!

1 Combine all herbs in a pot, and cover with boiling water.

2 Stir well, cover, and steep 15 to 20 minutes.

STEAMIN' MAMA'S LEMONADE

Juice of 1 lemon (organic)

1–2 tablespoons honey

⅛–¼ teaspoon cayenne pepper

Not for the timid or unadventurous! Okay, so it's not technically a tea, but worth its weight in gold when you've got a cold. Keep a box of tissues nearby, and be prepared to blow those germs away.

1 Squeeze the lemon into 2 cups boiling water, and add the honey and cayenne.

2 Stir well and sip slowly.

Garlic Ginger Tea

A powerful assault on flu bugs, this tea is guaranteed to knock germs out and probably knock your socks off too! The combination of ingredients might sound weird, but it actually tastes good! It's spicy, aromatic, and warming.

2 tablespoons ginger root, freshly grated

2 cloves of garlic, freshly crushed or chopped

4-5 fresh orange slices (organic)

Juice of 1 lemon (organic)

1-2 tablespoons honey

1 Add the ginger, garlic, and orange to 2 cups boiling water, reduce heat, and gently simmer for 5 to 10 minutes.

2 Turn off the heat, and steep 15 to 20 minutes.

3 Squeeze in the lemon juice, sweeten with honey, and get ready to blast off!

Hot Sweats Tea

From an old herbal diaphoretic formula, this is a tasty, spicy tea sure to make you sweat buckets!

1 part elder flowers

1 part ginger root, freshly grated

1 part peppermint leaves

Pinch of cayenne pepper

Juice of 1 lemon (organic)

1-2 tablespoons honey

1 Combine all herbs in a pot, and cover with boiling water.

2 Stir well, cover, and steep 15 to 20 minutes.

3 Add lemon and honey.

ANTIVIRAL SUPREME

½ **part ginger root, freshly grated**

1 **part rose hips (organic)**

1 **part sage leaves**

1 **part thyme leaves**

½ **part peppermint leaves**

1–2 **droppersful of echinacea and/or usnea tinctures***

*Available in health food stores

Take this unique and powerful antiviral, antibacterial tea three to five times per day for maximum benefit.

1. Add the ginger and rose hips to boiling water, reduce heat, and gently simmer for 5 to 10 minutes.

2. Turn off the heat, add the remaining herbs, and steep, covered, 15 to 20 minutes. Add the tinctures to the last few sips of the tea.

Earache Ease

¼ **cup olive oil**

4 **cloves of garlic, freshly crushed**

½ **teaspoon pure tea tree essential oil***

½ **teaspoon pure lavender essential oil***

*Available in health food stores.

The most effective approach to earaches involves treating the infection inside and out. Antiseptic herbal oils can be applied in the ear, while antibiotic herbal teas and tinctures can be utilized to fight the infection internally. This oil doesn't have a long shelf life, so discard it after one week. To use, gently warm 1 teaspoon at a time. Saturate half of a cotton ball with warm oil, and place in the ear canal. Use the other half of the cotton ball to hold the oil-drenched part in place. Wear overnight if necessary.

1. Put the olive oil in a small clean jar, then put the jar in a small saucepan filled with a few inches of water. Gently warm the oil.

2. Turn off the heat and add the crushed garlic. Stir, cover the jar and let it steep 1 to 2 hours.

3. Strain out the garlic and add the essential oils.

SNIFFLE BUSTER TEA

Delightful, aromatic, and medicinally correct, this tea is oh-so-useful in warding off the cold and flu blues.

1 Combine all herbs in a pot, and cover with boiling water.

2 Stir well, cover, and steep 15 to 20 minutes.

1 **part fennel (fresh leaves, stalks, flowers, and seeds, or dried seeds)**

1 **part ginger root, freshly grated**

1 **part rose hips (organic)**

1 **part sage leaves**

1 **part thyme leaves**

⅛ **part orange slices (organic)**

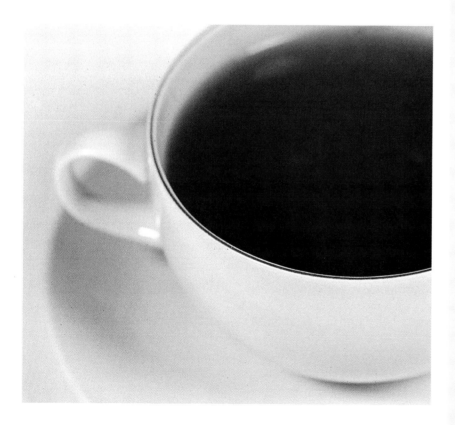

ALOHA
Barbara Fahs
San Jose, California

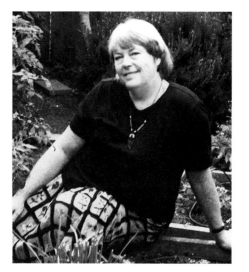

After a 28-year involvement with herbs, Barb Fahs is making her dream a reality. She's moving to Hawaii to establish an educational herb garden, produce and sell herbal products, and teach. After visiting a friend in Hawaii in 1981, Barb fell in love with the magic there and planned her eventual getaway.

Her journey started in 1971, when she started growing herbs for culinary use. She credits Brysis Buchanan of Santa Cruz for motivating her interest in herbs, which was sparked after going on a nature walk with Brysis. "I believe in taking care of myself and learning about herbs is an important part of acting on this goal," she says.

Barb also studied with Louis and Virginia Saso and remembers weeding their incredible gardens. Another pivotal experience, what she describes as "a highlight in her life," was visiting the Ix Chel Herb Farm in Belize in 1997. She says books by Rosita Arvigo and Michael Tierra are prominent on her shelves. Another milestone she cites is becoming a Master Gardener.

Born in England, Barb lived there with her American parents while her father was a foreign correspondent. She grew up in the San Francisco Bay area, attending the University of California at Santa Barbara to receive a degree in anthropology. Barb has worked as a technical writer for 14 years. "I see a dearth of values in the high-tech industry," she explains. "People are making themselves ill eating fast food, working too hard, driving too fast, stressing themselves out, and totally losing sight of the only thing that really matters: the earth and our continued success as residents of it." She hopes to educate people about how to take care of themselves and be happier, doing it in an earth-friendly manner.

She tells of an experience when, at the moment of learning that redwood trees have medicinal properties, she had a flash of enlightenment. "I realized that *all* plants have chemical properties that render them useful in some way," she exclaims, "either treating various conditions or in dyes, cosmetics, etc." Favorites in her pharmacopoeia include echinacea for its healing powers, catnip, which is good for colds, and chamomile, which is a sleep promoter. Her advice to those would-be tea makers out there: Experiment!

BARB'S COLD COMFORT

Barb swears by this remedy, stating this tea helped her recover quickly from a really bad cold. She recommends fresh herbs if possible, or good-quality dried herbs, adding that the tea is stronger because of the decoction process, rather than just steeping. "Drink a lot of it," Barb says, "but be aware that the yarrow can cause heat flushing, good for breaking a fever."

1 part echinacea root

1 part peppermint leaves

1 part catnip leaves

1 part yarrow leaves

1 part lemon balm leaves

❶ Put echinacea in 1 quart of water and bring to a boil. Simmer, covered, for 20 minutes.

❷ Add the rest of the herbs, stir well, cover and steep 15 to 20 minutes.

❸ Strain and add honey and lemon, if desired.

THE LADIES' ROOM

This section includes recipes addressing the events in life that are uniquely female. Personally, I wish I had known about PMS Blues-B-Gone Tea earlier in my life, as it probably would have made me saner sooner. I remember a male doctor telling me once (a long time ago) that there was so such thing as PMS. Hah! Ever feel like you gain about 20 pounds just before your period? I'm sure the Bloat Banishing formula can help with that problem, and there's a nourishing prenatal blend to support both mother and future blessing.

PMS BLUES-B-GONE TEA

1 part lemon balm leaves

1 part lemon verbena leaves

1 part nettle leaves

1 part oatstraw

1 part passiflora leaves

1 part St.-John's-wort flowers

Start drinking this blend about a week before menses. Gently toning, calming, and nourishing the nervous system, it helps alleviate common symptoms of PMS, such as moodiness and irritability.

1 Combine all herbs in a pot, and cover with boiling water.

2 Stir well, cover, and steep 15 to 20 minutes.

Herbal Diuretics

Not only are herbal diuretics generally safer than the commercial varieties, but they also provide a rich list of minerals, particularly potassium, which is commonly depleted by drugs that do the same job.

BLOAT-BANISHING NUTRIENT TEA

Besides offering high mineral content, this tea is a gentle and safe diuretic to help ease the weight gain associated with the premenstrual phase.

1 part dandelion root
1 part dandelion leaves
1 part horsetail
1 part nettle leaves
¼ part parsley leaves
½ part spearmint leaves

1 Add the dandelion root to boiling water, reduce heat, and simmer for 10 minutes in a covered pot.

2 Turn off the heat, and add the remaining ingredients.

3 Steep, covered, 15 to 20 minutes.

SOOTHING SPIRIT TEA

This delightfully uplifting tea tones the nerves and uterus and is good to drink during the premenstrual phase. Pre-, mid-, and post-menopausal women will also find it helpful. It's good tasting and good for your spirit. Men can enjoy it too.

1 part chamomile flowers
1 part linden flowers
1 part oatstraw
1 part passiflora leaves
1 part red raspberry leaves
¼ part orange slices (organic)
1/10 part lavender flowers (organic)
1/10 part rose petals (organic)
1/10 part jasmine flowers

1 Combine all herbs in a pot, and cover with boiling water.

2 Stir well, cover, and steep 15 to 20 minutes.

NURTURING PRENATAL BLEND

1 **part nettle leaves**

1 **part oatstraw**

1 **part red raspberry leaves**

1 **part rose hips (organic)**

1 **part spearmint leaves**

1 **part squaw vine leaves**

A mineral-rich blend, this tea is excellent for strengthening and preparing the uterus for childbearing. Drink it before and during pregnancy to help nourish nerves and bones.

1 Combine all herbs in a pot, and cover with boiling water.

2 Stir well, cover, and steep 15 to 20 minutes.

HERBAL IRON TONIC

1 **part nettle leaves**

1 **part oatstraw**

1 **part red raspberry leaves**

1 **part rose hips (organic)**

1 **part dried cherries**

1 **part dried apricots, raisins, or currants**

½ **part yellow dock root**

Blackstrap molasses*

Brandy

Raspberry vinegar**

Available in most health food stores.

**Available in most health food stores, or make your own using 1 cup crushed, fresh or frozen raspberries infused overnight in 2 cups white wine vinegar. Strain, and voila!*

Use this great tonic for blood-building during pre- and postnatal times and also during PMS and menopause. Make it once or twice a year, then imbibe several times a week as a blood-enriching, iron-and-mineral boost. It will keep for several months if refrigerated.

1 Add all herbs and fruits to boiling water (1 quart per 1 ounce of herbs), reduce heat, and simmer for 2 hours, covered.

2 Remove from the heat, and allow to steep 2 hours, covered.

3 Stir occasionally.

4 Strain out all the solids, squeezing all liquid through cheesecloth.

5 Measure the volume of tea, then add one-half to three-quarters as much molasses, ¼ part brandy (to preserve), and a couple of dashes of raspberry vinegar.

6 Keep refrigerated, taking 1 to 2 tablespoons as needed.

NOURISHING ENDOCRINE ELIXIR

Wonderful for balancing and strengthening the female being, this formula supports the hormonal and glandular systems. It's yummy and nourishing and can be made as a tea or tinctured in brandy. As a tea, drink 1 to 2 cups daily. As an elixir, take 1 to 2 dropperfuls two to four times per day.

1 **For tea:** Add all herbs to boiling water, reduce heat, and simmer for 15 to 20 minutes in a covered pot.

2 Turn off the heat, and steep, covered, 15 to 20 minutes.

3 **For elixir:** Simmer herbs 40 minutes, turn off the heat, and steep 20 minutes.

4 Strain, squeezing all the excess liquid from the herbs.

5 Measure the volume of the liquid, then add one-half to three-quarters as much molasses and ¼ part brandy.

1 **part dandelion root**

1 **part dong quai root**

1 **part cooked rehmannia root**

1 **part sarsaparilla root**

1 **part Siberian ginseng root**

Blackstrap molasses*

Brandy

Available in most health food stores.

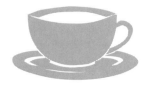

MOUNTAIN MAGIC
Shatoiya de la Tour
Auburn, California

Nestled in the scenic foothills of the Sierras, Dry Creek Herb Farm and Learning Center evolved from the dreams and visions of Shatoiya de la Tour, who was guided by the needs of her community and her determination to live independently off the land. Her relationship with herbs began some 30 years ago, with a 12-year period she describes as being taught solely by the plants. "We evolved with herbs," Shatoiya

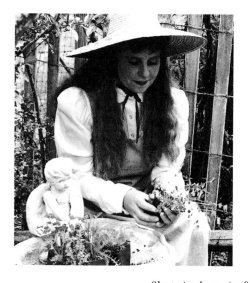

says. "They are our allies. We care for them in our garden and respect them in the wild and they, in turn, offer us their healing powers."

Besides her green teachers, she sought knowledge from herbal elders. "I hung out at the health food stores, talking to the old folks," she says, crediting mountain herbalist Marina Bokelman for teaching her the importance of humility. Shatoiya gained what she calls "a path of earth-centered spirituality" from her association with Rosemary Gladstar at the California School of Herbal Studies, then went on to establish Dry Creek Herb Farm, the two-acre display gardens, farm, and educational resource center lovingly tended with her husband, Rick.

Shatoiya's main focus is education, with apprenticeship programs, an ambitious menu of classes, events, workshops, and intensives. "Every day I give thanks that I earn my living doing what I love," she says. The paradise of Shatoiya's gardens is a living testimony to this love. "It's my goal that people visiting our gardens be touched by the beauty and realize that nature provides for our healing." Further blessings from Shatoiya's considerable wisdom and wit may be found in *Herbalist of Yarrow,* a charming fairy tale of the plant world she's written for both children and adult enjoyment.

"The primary service in our shop is custom-blending teas and tinctures," Shatoiya states. She's developed 25 basic tea blends, which she often uses as the base teas for her customer's special needs. "Teas are my favorite way to recommend herbs for health and pleasure. It's the best way to get the most of what an herb has to offer." She says the calming effect of ritual tea making, the full flavor on the tongue, and warmth in the throat are very natural and healing.

Her advice for people new to herbal tea: "Keep it simple and make sure it tastes good." She explains that infusions are easier for most people to make and urges you to use the highest quality of organically grown herbs available.

SHATOIYA'S MOON BREW

This tea contains simple, nutritive herbs and is great hot or iced. Although used regularly in her women's moon lodge ceremonies, Shatoiya recommends it for men as well.

● Use 1 teaspoon herbs per cup of water. Pour boiling water over herbs in a pot and steep, covered, 15 minutes or more.

1¼ parts raspberry leaves

1 part nettle leaves

½ part lavender flowers (organic)

½ part spearmint leaves

½ part rose petals (organic)

¼ part oatstraw

THE MANLY MAN

Hey, you men out there, think drinking a cup of herbal tea is not the most macho thing in the world to do and that it won't enhance your masculine image? Well, think again. Women will love you for it! And you'll be way ahead of the other guys because you'll be nourishing your heart and toning assorted other body parts.

GINSENG SWING

2 parts Siberian ginseng root

1 part dandelion root

1 part hawthorn berries

1 part sarsaparilla root

⅛ part cinnamon chips

¹⁄₁₀ part licorice root

¹⁄₁₀ part orange peel (organic)

Here's a great tonic for overall energy, stamina, and mental clarity. The hawthorn nourishes the heart, the dandelion tones the liver and digestive system, and the ginseng, sarsaparilla, and licorice nourish the adrenals and male glandular system. This makes a delicious tincture or elixir as well as tea. For instructions on making tinctures and elixirs, check out the information in the brewing chapter, pages 10–12. Drink ½ cup twice per day.

1 Add all herbs to boiling water, reduce heat, and simmer in a covered pot for 20 minutes.

2 Remove from the heat and steep, covered, 30 minutes.

Mr. Irresistibili-Tea

A delicious blend to enhance, romance, excite, and delight you!

1. Combine all herbs and cover with boiling water.

2. Stir well, cover, and steep 15 to 20 minutes.

3. Sweeten lightly with honey, if desired, and drink hot or cold.

4. Add candlelight and good music . . . and see what happens!

2 parts damiana leaves

1 part lemongrass leaves

1 part passiflora leaves

½ part spearmint leaves

¼ part jasmine flowers

⅛ part orange peel (organic)

1/10 part cinnamon chips

1/10 part lavender flowers (organic)

1/10 part rose petals (organic)

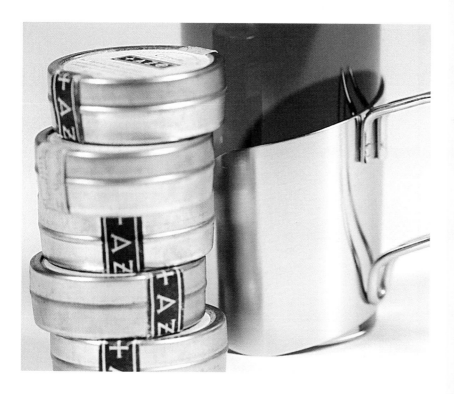

HEART SHAPED

The heart is such an important body part that it has its own day in mid-February, and commercial retailers make the most of it selling cards, gifts, and dinners out with your significant other. It's also probably the body part appearing most often in literature, songs, advertisements, and the like. But consider the real thing, our wonderful "ticker," that pulsating, midchest machine that deals us out each minute of every day. We all want to keep our heart in good shape, and here are several good ways to ensure that happens.

HEALTHY HEART'S DESIRE

3 parts hawthorn leaves and flowers

2 parts hawthorn berries

2 parts rose hips (organic)

1 part oatstraw

½ part linden blossoms

¼ part orange slices (organic)

This gentle, bioflavonoid-rich blend is wonderfully supportive when you are recovering from any kind of injury or surgery, nourishing the heart and cardiovascular system. It can be made into a superb elixir as well (see the instructions for making an elixir in the brewing chapter, page 12).

1 Combine all herbs in a pot, and cover with boiling water.

2 Stir well, cover, and steep 15 to 20 minutes.

3 Sweeten lightly with honey, if desired, and drink hot or cold.

Caution
Always seek qualified medical help in diagnosis and treatment of any medical condition.

Heart's Ease Tea

An excellent tea for relaxing and nourishing the heart and cardiovascular system, this formula is particularly valuable in easing angina. Hawthorn and ginkgo provide cardio-tonic flavonoids, and motherwort brings cardio-active glycosides to the blend. In addition, motherwort, linden, oatstraw, and crampbark have relaxing and antispasmodic properties that work wonderfully with hawthorn and ginkgo to aid a "stressed-out" heart. The violet leaf and flower are added for their nourishing vitamin and mineral content and for their beautiful heart-shaped leaves. Violets have, since ancient times, been affectionately known as "heart's ease." Drink 2 to 3 cups per day.

1 Combine all herbs in a pot, and cover with boiling water.

2 Stir well, cover, and steep 15 to 20 minutes.

3 **parts hawthorn leaves and flowers**

2 **parts hawthorn berries**

2 **parts ginkgo leaves**

2 **parts motherwort leaves**

2 **parts oatstraw**

2 **parts violet leaves and flowers**

1 **part crampbark**

1 **part linden blossoms**

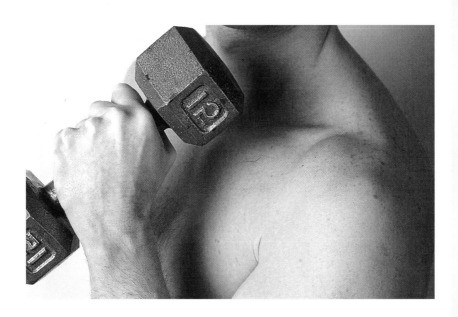

HEARTTHROB CORDIAL

1 part rose hips (organic)

1 part raspberries (fresh or frozen)

1 part hawthorn berries

Brandy

Both pretty and delicious, this blend is wonderful for the Christmas holidays and, as a bonus, good for the circulatory system. This would make an incredibly thoughtful gift, as you are not only giving a tasty brew but a sincere wish for continued good health as well. Take 1 to 2 tablespoons per day.

1. Cover herbs with three times as much brandy in a wide-mouthed jar, and cap tightly.

2. Shake daily for two to four weeks.

3. Strain, sweeten lightly with honey, and put in a pretty bottle.

HEART REVIVAL TEA

2 parts hawthorn berries

2 parts Siberian ginseng root

3 parts hawthorn leaves and flowers

2 parts ginkgo leaves

1 part linden blossoms

1 part nettle leaves

1 part rose hips (organic)

This nourishing formula has the classic tonic actions of hawthorn, combined with the strengthening properties of rose hips and ginkgo. Siberian ginseng safely helps the body adapt to stress and strengthens adrenal and glandular body functions. Nettle is one of the best blood and adrenal nourishers, rich in chlorophyll, beta-carotene, vitamin C, and iron. This gentle, yet effective, strengthening tea for overall heart health can be used by anyone who is recovering from a heart attack.

1. Add the hawthorn berries and ginseng root to boiling water, reduce heat, and simmer for 20 minutes in a covered pot.

2. Remove from the heat and add remaining herbs.

3. Steep, covered 15 to 20 minutes.

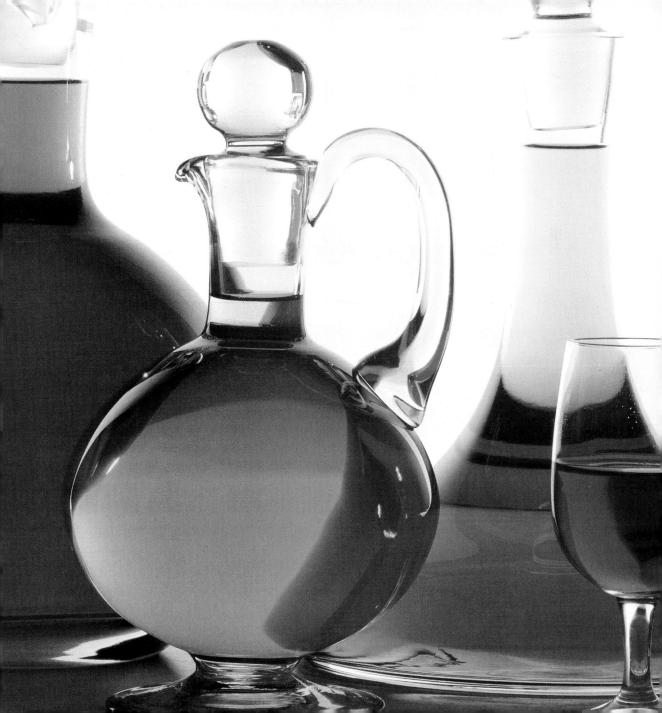

Skin Deep

Usually what's appearing on your face (oh, no, it's a zit!) is a reflection of what's going on inside your body. For teens, it's probably hormonal, but that doesn't mean the situation is hopeless. Skin problems at any age usually signal that it's time to deploy the heavy artillery, in this case, blood-purifying herbal teas that will address the problem, not the exterior manifestation. We've got a wonderful assortment of goodies for you in this section, including teas and a to-die-for toner that's so easy to make, we guarantee you'll never buy commercial toners again!

Five-Root Revival

1 part burdock root

1 part dandelion root

1 part sarsaparilla root

1 part yellow dock root

¼ part sassafras root bark

Traditionally, these roots were brewed into old-fashioned root beer and imbibed as a healthful liver- and blood-cleansing beverage. Drink 1 to 2 cups per day for mild to moderate skin problems. This makes a great tincture in brandy, too. There's information on how to make tinctures in the brewing chapter, pages 10–11.

❶ Combine all herbs in boiling water, reduce heat, and simmer for 15 to 20 minutes in a covered pot.

❷ Remove from the heat, and steep, covered, 30 minutes.

ZIT-AWAY TEA

Specifically for chronic or stubborn acne, this formula is cleansing to the lymph system, liver, and blood. Drink 2 to 4 cups per day for two to four weeks.

1 Add all herbs to boiling water, reduce heat, and simmer for 15 to 20 minutes in a covered pot.

2 Remove from the heat, and steep, covered, 30 minutes.

2 **parts echinacea root**

2 **parts redroot**

1 **part burdock root**

1 **part fresh dandelion root**

1 **part roasted dandelion root**

1 **part sarsaparilla root**

½ **part Oregon grape root**

Flower Power Facial Toner — for External Use Only!

1 **cup pure distilled rose water***

1 **cup pure distilled orange blossom water***

1 **cup distilled witch hazel**

½ **cup shredded fresh lavender and/or rose geranium blossoms (organic).**

¼ **cup aloe vera juice****

3 **drops pure lavender, rose geranium, or rose essential oil****

*Available in health food stores, herb shops, or Greek delis!
**Available in most health food stores.

Just think, now you can make your own refreshing and health enhancing toners. This is fantastic stuff — mildly astringent, soothing, and antiseptic. Apply after washing your face and also in between washings. Keep it in the refrigerator.

1 Place the first four ingredients in a clean, widemouthed glass jar.

2 Cap tightly, then shake well, and place in a sunny spot for 3 to 4 hours. Strain the herbs, pressing all the liquid out. Add the aloe vera and essential oil.

BREATHE EASY

You can hear that nasty congestion deep in your chest, rattling around, and it hurts to inhale deeply. It's miserable trying to sleep because it always seems to get worse at night, when you're lying down. Or, how about all that pollen? It's allergy season and your body is sinus challenged. All common ailments, and truly supported by what we've got for you below. The teas are incredible, and we've included an inhale that will really break up the congestion.

DECONGEST & FEEL YOUR BEST TEA

2 parts yerba santa leaves

2 parts sage leaves

1 part ginger root, freshly grated

1 part nettle leaves

1 part peppermint leaves

⅛ part licorice root

This is an excellent formula for congested, drippy sinuses due to colds or allergies. The yerba santa, nettle, and sage in combination gently help to dry up excess mucus in the upper respiratory tract, without the "overdrying" effect of many antihistamines. Sip freely as needed.

1 Combine all herbs in a pot, and cover with boiling water.

2 Stir well, cover, and steep 15 to 20 minutes.

Caution
There are several kinds of ephedra available. The Chinese ephedra (*Ephedra sinica*), known as *ma huang* contains alkaloids that are similar to adrenaline and can stimulate your heart rate and blood pressure. Use the western ephedra *(E. viridis)*, not *ma huang*, for the following recipe.

GET RID OF THE DRIP TEA

When your sinuses are driving you crazy, this tea is a godsend! It's a gentle tonic and anti-inflammatory to the nasal passages. Drink 2 cups per day about three to four weeks before allergy season begins its torture treatment. This allows the formula time to start working in advance of the actual onslaught of pollens and other springtime allergens.

2 parts elder flowers

1 part ephedra leaves

1 part goldenrod leaves

1 part nettle leaves

1. Combine all herbs in a pot, and cover with boiling water.

2. Stir well, cover, and steep 15 to 20 minutes.

In-hale and Hearty

If there is an acute sinus or bronchial infection present, supplement your healing tea regimen with this antiseptic herbal inhalation and treatment with supportive tinctures such as echinacea and usnea.

1. Add 2 handfuls of herbs from the list at right to 2 quarts boiled water. Cover and steep 1 minute.

2. Grab a large towel, sit down at a table, and lift cover off the pot. Add 1 or 2 drops of both eucalyptus and lavender essential oils, and, if the infection is persistent, add 2 drops each of tea tree and thyme essential oils as well.

3. Make a tent over both your head and the pan, and inhale. If you cough, the mixture is probably too strong, so vent the towel for a few seconds and resume.

HERBS TO USE FOR INHALATION AND BATHS

CALENDULA

CHAMOMILE

CITRUS PEELS

LAVENDER

LEMONGRASS

MINT

ROSE

ROSEMARY

SAGE

THYME

The Senior Advantage

Being in my middle years now, I feel qualified to say that getting older is actually not bad. I've come to embrace the wisdom the years and experiences have brought and honestly wouldn't go back to relive my tumultuous youth (except, of course, if I could go back knowing what I know now!). But, let's face it, there are health issues to face at this time of life that are usually unique to the more "experienced adults." The following blends are not only helpful in coming to terms with, for instance, keeping your bones strong, but are delicious and easy to make.

Strong Bones Tea

2 parts oatstraw

1 part alfalfa leaves

1 part horsetail

1 part red clover blossoms

1 part rose hips (organic)

1 part violet leaves and flowers

2 parts nettle

Here's a blend that gently provides minerals for the entire body. All these herbs are nutritious and tend to be good sources of absorbable calcium, magnesium, iron, and other important trace minerals. Drink 2 to 4 cups per day as a gentle bone-building tonic.

1 Combine all herbs in a pot, and cover with boiling water.

2 Stir well, cover, and steep 15 to 20 minutes.

SHOUT OUT GOUT TEA

To help flush excess uric acid deposits out of the body, use this gentle alkalizing blend. Drink 3 to 4 cups of the tea daily as a preventive measure.

1. Combine all herbs in a pot, and cover with boiling water.

2. Stir well, cover, and steep 15 to 20 minutes.

2 **parts nettle leaves**

1 **part alfalfa leaves**

1 **part celery seeds**

1 **part dandelion leaves**

1 **part dandelion root**

1 **part oatstraw**

HEART & SOUL TONIC

Rich in beta-carotene and bioflavonoids, this yummy raspberry-based cordial is a true tonic that's fun to take. It increases circulation to and from the heart and brain and increases the integrity of tissues and capillaries, making it excellent for people who bruise easily and heal slowly. It's useful as a pre- and postsurgery tonic and helpful in healing any structural injury to bones, ligaments, tendons, and muscles. Take ½ teaspoon once or twice a day, three to five times a week, or daily for the two-week periods before and after surgery. If you'd prefer the wonderful tonic qualities as a tea, steep the ingredients (except the raspberries) in 1 quart boiled water 15 to 20 minutes in a covered pot. Drink 1 or 2 cups per day.

● Grind all the herbs and place in a widemouthed jar, then cover with three times as much brandy. Let it stand one month, then strain, squeezing all liquid from the herbs. Sweeten with honey.

2 **parts ginkgo leaves**

2 **parts hawthorn flowers and leaves**

2 **parts hawthorn berries**

1 **part orange slices (organic)**

1 **part raspberries (fresh or frozen)**

1 **part rose hips (organic)**

2 **tablespoons honey (per pint of strained liquid)**

Brandy

THE TERRIBLE TEENS

Okay, it's that up-and-down time of life when you're questioning who you are today, who you'll be tomorrow, and what you're going to be when you grow up — something every person on the planet has experienced or will experience at one time or another, usually during, but not limited to, the teen years. Your hormones are really the issue in the terrible teens, but they do eventually stop screaming. What you really want is to *survive* this phase of life and to get rid of that pimple before your prom, first date, cheerleading tryouts, or whatever. The formulas below help with the zits and other issues at stake. By the way, these blends are good for the post-teenagers, too, who might still be wondering who they're going to be when they grow up, and may even still get oh-no zits!

HORMONE HELPER

2 parts sarsaparilla root

2 parts Siberian ginseng root

1 part dandelion root

1 part oatstraw

1 part vitex berries

Appropriate for both sexes, this earthy, rooty blend supports the liver and glandular system and helps balance hormones. Drink 2 to 4 cups per day, four to five times per week. Since teens may resist drinking herbal teas, this formula can be tinctured (see directions for making tinctures in the brewing chapter, pages 10–11). Take ½ to 1 teaspoon of tincture twice a day, five days a week.

❶ Combine all herbs boiling water, reduce heat, and simmer for 20 minutes in a covered pot.

❷ Remove from the heat and steep, covered, 20 minutes.

Raging Moods Tea

Hot or iced, this tea is particularly good for those unexpected, unwanted, and stubborn mood swings. Drink 2 to 4 cups per day when you feel your moods and/or hormones running amok.

2 parts oatstraw

2 parts skullcap leaves

1 part passiflora leaves

1 part St.-John's-wort flowers

½ part spearmint leaves

⅒ part lavender flowers (organic)

1. Combine all herbs in a pot, and cover with boiling water.

2. Stir well, cover, and steep 15 to 20 minutes.

3. Sweeten lightly with honey, if desired.

A Pimple's Worst Nightmare Tea

Use this bitter brew to help cleanse the liver and blood, clear the skin, and make your zits reevaluate their decision to inhabit your body! Drink 2 to 4 cups per day, four or five times a week. This is another blend that can be tinctured (see the information on making tinctures in the brewing chapter on pages 10–11). Take ½ to 1 teaspoon of tincture twice a day, five days a week.

1 part burdock root

1 part dandelion root

1 part echinacea root

1 part Oregon grape root

1 part yellow dock root

1 part sarsaparilla

1. Add all roots to boiling water, reduce heat, and simmer for 20 minutes in a covered pot.

2. Remove from the heat, and steep, covered, 20 minutes.

Face Off

There are all sorts of changes going on inside a teen's body, and the outside image reflects this. And isn't it always the way that just when you're going on that special date or some equally important event, here comes a zit, or a whole parade of them? This quick steam and masque are good ways to deeply cleanse, nourish, and tone your skin. It smells and feels wonderful. Once a week is optimum.

QUICK PRE-MASQUE STEAMER

1-2 drops pure lavender or rose geranium essential oil*

Add 1 or 2 drops of pure lavender or rose geranium essential oil to 1 quart of comfortably hot water. Stir well, then dip a clean washcloth into the water. Squeeze out the excess water, close your eyes, and lay the cloth over your face. As the cloth cools, redip and repeat the process for 2 to 3 minutes. Follow up with the masque.

OH NO! IT'S A ZIT ATTACK MASQUE

1 teaspoon green clay*

1 teaspoon honey

1 teaspoon peach or apricot yogurt

1 drop pure lavender or rose geranium essential oil*

Available at most health food stores.

Mix the first three ingredients well, then add the essential oil. Spread the mixture on your face, lie down, and relax for 15 to 30 minutes. The masque won't stiffen completely due to the yogurt and honey. Rinse with warm water, and use a washcloth to gently remove the goop. Splash with cool water afterward.

OPPORTUNITY KNOCKS
Lynda Lewit, *Soquel, California*

As a public health nurse for Children's Protective Services, Lynda Lewit has a unique opportunity to introduce the benefits of herbs to others. She is quick to note that she always works in combination with allopathic doctors in suggesting herbal remedies, but she finds that more and more frequently, even those icons of the medical profession are open to alternative methods that herbs provide. Though she makes many herbal products herself, Lynda suggests commercial teas and tinctures for the foster children whose health she helps to oversee, treating such chronic health issues as upper respiratory infections and ear problems. Lynda also suggests complementary herbal therapies which aid in her young patient's preventive care. Lynda enjoys teaching and always prepares herbal teas for her foster parent meetings, and finds the parents are interested in teas and herbal baths that help them relax.

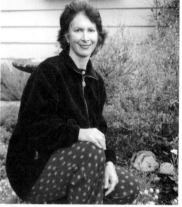

Her advice to those wishing to gain more plant knowledge is be patient when learning about herbs and be respectful of the plants. Lynda adds a caution for would-be wildcrafters: "Be 100 percent sure of the plants you're picking in the fields."

DIVA'S PMS BE GONE TEA

This mineral-rich tea has a diuretic effect and is calming to the nerves. Drink 1 to 2 cups per day of this healthy, earthy-tasting blend.

2 parts nettle leaves

1 part apple mint or lemon balm leaves

1 part lemon verbena leaves

● Add herbs to boiling water, steep, covered, 20 minutes. Drink hot or cool, for the three days prior to menstruation.

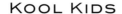

KOOL KIDS

Be the first kid on your block to tout the benefits of herbal tea. You can set up a sidewalk stand and sell herbal teas to all who pass. Tell your friends how well the Yummy-Tummy Tea works after eating too much junk food, then set up a booth in your yard that says "The Doctor Is In." Or better yet, I'll bet all the moms on your block will pay good money for the Kiddie Calm recipe.

KIDDIE CALM

2 **parts chamomile flowers**

1 **part catnip leaves**

1 **part lemon balm leaves**

1 **part oatstraw**

This gentle, safe, and calming blend is specific for little ones who are restless or over-excited. For babies, you can put this tea in their bottles or give it to them by the dropperful or teaspoonful 3 times per day. Older children, for example 6 to 10 years old, may have ¼ to ½ cup 3 times per day.

1 Combine all herbs in a pot, and cover with boiling water.

2 Stir well, cover, and steep 15 to 20 minutes.

KIDDIE COLD-CHASER TEA

A tasty antiviral blend that fights off colds, this tea also calms the tummy and nerves. Give it to babies in their bottles, or by the teaspoon or dropperful 3 times a day. For older children ¼ to ½ cup 3 times a day is given. It tastes so good that even "big kids" will enjoy it!

1 Combine all herbs in a pot, and cover with boiling water.

2 Stir well, cover, and steep 15 to 20 minutes.

3 Strain and add fresh lemon juice and honey.

2 parts lemon balm leaves

1 part catnip leaves

1 part elder flowers

1 part fennel (fresh leaves and stalks or dried seeds)

1 part rose hips (organic)

¼ part ginger root, freshly grated

Lemon juice and honey, to taste

TERRIFIC YUMMY-TUMMY TEA

Great for upset tummies and even stomach flu, this tea is soothing and tastes wonderful, for kids of all ages! Give little sips until relief is obtained.

1 Combine all herbs in a pot, and cover with boiling water.

2 Stir well, cover, and steep 15 to 20 minutes.

1 part peppermint leaves

1 part spearmint leaves

½ part anise or fennel seeds

⅛ part licorice root

⅛ part orange or tangerine slices (organic)

The Uplifters

Your canary just died, you just got a notice from the IRS that you're being audited, *and* your kids put your wool sweater in the dryer. On the high setting. You're low. Make tea. You leave for work and your tire's flat. In the snow. Follow these simple instructions: Return to the house, call for roadside assistance, drink a cup of Happy Spirits in therapeutic sips. Give a cup to the tow truck driver when he arrives. Pass go and start again. And for those more lengthy troughs in life, I definitely recommend the Lift Off special.

Euphoria Tea

1 part fennel (fresh leaves and stalks)

1 part lemon verbena leaves

1 part rose geranium leaves and flowers (organic)

A fragrant, uplifting blend that's sure to become a summer favorite. It's best made from fresh herbs, but dried will do. Serve hot or iced.

❶ Combine all herbs in a pot, and cover with boiling water.

❷ Stir well, cover, and steep 15 to 20 minutes.

❸ Serve with a little honey, if desired.

Happy Spirits Tea

2 parts lemon balm leaves

2 parts lemon verbena leaves

1 part catnip leaves

1 part oatstraw

1 part passiflora leaves

¼ part tangerine slices (organic)

¹⁄₁₀ part cinnamon chips

No matter how bad things look, this tea will ease your woes. We guarantee things will start to look up after sipping this gently nourishing blend.

❶ Combine all herbs in a pot, and cover with boiling water.

❷ Stir well, cover, and steep 15 to 20 minutes.

LIFT OFF

For times of stress, worry, and anxiety, this tea soothes even the most frazzled nerves while, what else, lifting the spirits waaaaay up.

1. Combine all herbs in a pot, and cover with boiling water.

2. Stir well, cover, and steep 15 to 20 minutes.

3. Add the tincture to the last few sips of tea, up to three times per day.

1 part chamomile flowers

1 part hawthorn flowers, leaves, and berries

1 part lemon balm leaves

1 part oatstraw

1 part St.-John's-wort flowers

1 part skullcap leaves

⅛ part lavender flowers (organic)

1–2 dropperfuls Siberian ginseng tincture*

ANXIETY B-GONE

This tea is really for that type of depression where anxiety is rearing its ugly head.

1. Combine all herbs in a pot, and cover with boiling water.

2. Stir well, cover, and steep 15 to 20 minutes.

3. Add the tincture to the last few sips of tea, up to four times per day.

1 part chamomile flowers

1 part lemon verbena leaves

1 part oatstraw

1 part passiflora leaves

1 part skullcap leaves

1–2 dropperfuls valerian/wild poppy tincture*

*Available in health food stores.

DYNAMIC DUO
Madelene Hill & Gwen Barclay
Round Top, Texas

This mother-daughter team, both proud native Texans, has made herbs a daily part of their lives. Gwen Barclay is the Director of Food Services at the International Festival Institute in Round Top, an impressive 210-acre facility devoted to musical, and often herbal, study. She plans all the meals, events, and educational activities. Madelene Hill, her mother, is the curator of the McAshon herb garden there.

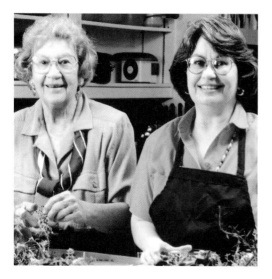

Madelene grew up with herbs as a child in Kansas, living in German and Dutch communities for whom herb usage was a way of life. She credits this early life for her lifelong interest in plants and describes herself as a frustrated botanist. "I wish I had pursued an academic degree (in botany), but as the oldest of 13 children, that wasn't possible," she says. Instead, she has studied on her own, building an extensive reference library.

Gwen credits her mother for her herbal inspiration, describing her as " a phenomenal source of plant information and a memory to go with it." Gwen also recognizes Dr. Art Tucker of Delaware State University for his generosity of both expertise and time, explaining this is typical of the way most people in the herb industry share information.

After they retired, Madelene, with her husband, Jim, decided to take on the daunting task of growing gladiolus and planted an herb garden at the same time. Ten years later, they established Hilltop Herb Farm in the Houston area. Gwen joined the team in 1972, and they were among the first to offer fresh-cut herbs, dressings, butters, chutneys, and jalapeño jellies to the Houston restaurant industry. In 1983 a tornado destroyed the entire Hilltop operation, just as 100 guests were arriving for dinner.

After a decade of traveling, teaching, and sharing their vast knowledge and experience, mother and daughter landed at Round Top. They both enjoy meeting and teaching people about herbs. Together they have coauthored the popular book *Southern Herb Growing.*

Madelene and Gwen use herbal teas more for pleasure than medicine, but support research to identify accurate information about therapeutic benefits. They caution all tea makers to be careful about self-diagnosis and more importantly, to deal only with the botanical names in identifying the herbs to be used, not common names, which can vary greatly by region and lore.

MADELENE & GWEN'S FESTIVI-TEA

This delicious tea is a staple at the Festival Institute, one which any visitor to their events and classes will have sampled (repeatedly!). Madelene and Gwen say it may be combined with black China tea and served hot or iced.

● Pour boiling water over the herbs and steep 10 to 15 minutes in a covered pot.

- 1 part peppermint leaves
- 1 part chamomile flowers
- 1 part linden blossoms
- 1 part spearmint leaves
- 1 part rose hips (organic), crushed
- 1 part lemon verbena leaves
- 1 part lemon balm leaves

Work Out!

For you jocks and jockettes out there in fitness land, these teas are just the ticket. Amaze and astound your friends with feats of strength and stamina. When you tell them it's all because of your herbal tea, they will admire and respect your mental as well as physical prowess. Just do it.

Flexibility Tea

2 parts oatstraw

2 parts horsetail

1 part alfalfa leaves

1 part hawthorn berries, crushed

1 part red clover blossoms

1 part rose hips (organic)

¼ part orange slices (organic)

Nutrient rich, this blend helps nourish the ligaments, bones, joints, and tendons. It's a great recipe for sports injury recovery and pre- and post-surgery. Drink up to 4 cups per day, hot or iced.

❶ Combine all herbs in a pot, and cover with boiling water.

❷ Stir well, cover, and steep 15 to 20 minutes.

STRENGTH & STAMINA TEA

Let this hearty and very tasty tea assist your metabolism, cellular respiration, and liver — all factors that play a part in aerobic exercise. Drink 1 cup before working out. It's also excellent tinctured in brandy (see the information on making tinctures in the brewing section, pages 10–11). Let the tincture sit from one to three months before straining and imbibing.

2 parts Siberian ginseng root

2 parts Korean Red or Chinese Red ginseng root

1 part raw dandelion root

1 part roasted dandelion root

1 part sarsaparilla root

1/10 part ginger root, freshly grated

1/10 part cinnamon chips

1 Add approximately 1 ounce of herb blend to 1 quart of boiling water, reduce heat, and simmer for 30 minutes in a covered pot.

2 Turn off the heat, and steep 30 minutes.

Caution

Korean Red and Chinese Red ginsengs are strong tonics and should not be used by anyone who has a history of high blood pressure or heart palpitations. Siberian ginseng, however, is considered safe for these conditions, so just leave out the Korean Red or Chinese Red ginseng when making Strength & Stamina Tea.

A BLAZING STAR
Gail Ulrich
Shelburne Falls, Massachusetts

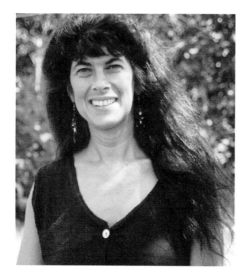

Although Gail Ulrich has been interested in herbs since child-hood, she began studying in earnest in the early 1970s when she found relief from health problems through herbal therapy. After suffering from cystitis for more than 10 years, she was able to relieve all symptoms in a matter of weeks by drinking a simple tea of nettles and corn silk. "Once you become involved with herbs," Gail says, "it changes your whole life and the lives of all those you touch." She names her chiropractor father, Dr. S. S. Ulrich, and country herbalist Delima Remo as her mentors and espe-cially thanks Doug Elliot for introducing her to the plants of the Blue Ridge Mountains.

Among the many impressive milestones on Gail's herbal path, she includes starting her Blaz-ing Star Herbal School in 1983 and creating a line of herbal products called New England Botanicals in 1984 as her most cherished. She pioneered the New England Women's Herbal Conference in 1987 and was cofounder of the Healing with Flowers Conference as well. In addition to being vice pres-ident of the Northeast Herbal Association, she's done formulas for Frontier Herbs and Estelle Hummel's line called Tasha's Herbs for Dogs. A popular teacher and speaker at conferences throughout the country, Gail also writes about herbs, including a book entitled *Herbs to Boost Immunity.*

Gail believes that herbal teas are an excellent way to benefit from the water-soluble constituents of plants. "They are a simple and time-honored way to nurture and take care of oneself," she explains. Her advice for tea-makers-in-training: Choose herbs that taste good. "Herbs with strong or unpleasant flavors are best used in tinctures or capsules."

"Decide what you wish to achieve with your tea," she suggests, a soothing, tasty beverage or a medicinal brew. If using teas therapeutically, she suggests keeping it simple. "Complex combinations can be difficult to blend, ending up with a muddy-tasting combination," she says. "There is no substitute for quality. Your herbal teas or preparations will only be as good as the herbs you put in." She advises buying organic herbs from reputable sources that are fresh and aromatic. The enlivening qualities of peppermint rank high on Gail's list of favorites, along with lemon balm for its soothing properties in treating nerve-related disorders and fennel, which she says is great for kids.

With the resurgence of interest in herbs comes an important need for good herbal education, Gail believes, so that herbal self-care can be implemented with safety and efficacy. "The herbal world is definitely my passion," says Gail. "I can't imagine any other lifestyle."

GAIL'S HIGH-CALCIUM TEA

A safe blend for improving calcium levels, this is excellent for women who wish to prevent osteoporosis, as well as those who want to relieve menstrual cramps, heal from broken bones, and improve teeth and gum health.

⬤ Combine all herbs in a pot. Cover with boiling water, stir well, cover and steep 10 to 20 minutes.

2 parts red raspberry leaves

2 parts red clover blossoms

2 parts nettle leaves

1 part lemon balm leaves

1 part peppermint leaves

1 part spearmint leaves

½ part calendula flowers

½ part lemon verbena leaves

½ part rose petals

SENSE & SENSIBILITY

Who hasn't been in a situation where real brainpower was required — at work, school, or just impressing your friends with flashes of brilliance. In this section, we've got just the thing to get those synapses snapping. After drinking If Only I Had a Brain Tea, you will probably win the Nobel prize or, at the very least, applaud yourself for doing such a smart thing as drinking it in the first place. Maybe you've got a really hot date and, while all the props are in place, you need a little "propping up" yourself. You're anxious, you're restless, you know the signs. The Moon Lightening blend can prove illuminating! These teas are sense-sational!

MOON LIGHTENING TEA

2 parts damiana leaves

1 part chamomile flowers

1 part lemongrass leaves

1 part oatstraw

1 part peppermint leaves

1 part rose hips (organic)

¼ part jasmine flowers

¼ part orange or tangerine slices (organic)

⅛ part lavender flowers (organic)

A colorful and flavorful blend for enhancing those cozy, romantic events, this tea is exotic and delectable. Need we say more?

1 Combine all herbs in a pot, and cover with boiling water.

2 Stir well, cover, and steep 15 to 20 minutes.

IF ONLY I HAD A BRAIN TEA

When you have to study, write, or think brilliant thoughts, this tea is great for mental clarity. Drink 2 or 3 cups per day. It also makes a nice-tasting tincture in brandy. (See the information on making tinctures in the brewing section, pages 10–11.)

2 parts Siberian ginseng root

1 part ginkgo leaves

1 part gotu kola leaves

1 part peppermint

1. Add the ginseng root to boiling water, reduce heat, and simmer in a covered pot for 20 minutes.

2. Turn off the heat, add the remaining herbs, and steep 20 minutes.

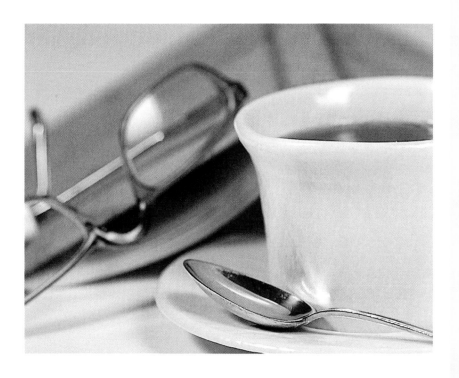

WELL GROUNDED
Kathi Keville
Nevada City, California

Kathi Keville is prolific in sharing her considerable herbal knowledge, and her name is well respected as herbalist, author, teacher, aromatherapist, and masseuse. After spending the past 30 years working with medicinal herbs, she is the highly qualified author of 10 books and more than 150 articles on herbs. In addition to her writing, Kathi has taught seminars from coast to coast and been involved in literature and product

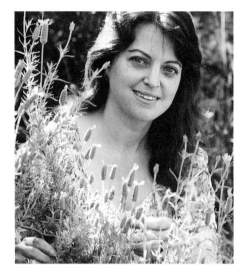

development. Her credentials include the position of Director of the American Herb Association, editor of their quarterly newsletter, and founding and honorary member of both the American Herbalists Guild and National Association of Holistic Aromatherapy.

Kathi's herbal knowledge is well grounded. She first became interested in herbs by growing them in her garden and gives much credit to the plants themselves for teaching her what she knows. "I realized my herb garden contained an entire pharmacopoeia of medicinal plants," she says. After owning and managing the Oak Valley Herb Farm for 15 years, including a 400-species herb garden, she now owns a mail-order herb and aromatherapy company by the same name.

Herb teas warm the body and soul on a cool, winter day or cool the heat of summer, Kathi believes. "It offers time for contemplation and a healthy dose of emotional and physical well-being," she adds. "Tasting the herb and inhaling the aroma enhance assimilation, too."

She recommends herbal tea as a great way to familiarize yourself with herbs, even if therapeutic results are not your initial goals. If and when they are, however, Kathi believes that "many ailments have responded amazingly well to tea, and that it's an excellent way to take your medicine!" Additionally, she feels that the tea making itself is a valuable part of the healing process. "There are benefits from simply sitting down and relaxing long enough to sip tea, often neglected in this fast-paced world."

An interesting variation Kathi suggests to herbal tea is herbal punch — combining your favorite herbal tea with an equal amount of fruit juice. For extra spirit, she adds a carbonated herbal soda to fruit juice. Another novel idea from Kathi is herbal ice cubes! She suggests freezing herbal teas into ice cubes, making them extra fancy by putting a sprig, leaf, or flower into the cube before freezing. She goes on from there to offer the idea of herbal Popsicles for kids (and adults, too). "Hibiscus is a favorite ingredient since it turns the Popsicle red," she adds.

KATHI'S TROPICAL TEA

Keep cool in the summer and take pleasure in knowing this blend is healthful as well as tasty! (Please note that the equivalent in this recipe for "part" is 3 tablespoons.)

1 part hibiscus flowers

1 part mint leaves

1 part lemongrass leaves

½ cup chopped pineapple

2 oranges (organic), sliced

1 papaya, sliced

1 mango, sliced (or other tropical fruit)

1 Bring 2 quarts water to a boil, turn off the heat, and add the herbs. Steep, covered, 20 minutes and strain.

2 Put fruit into a 2-quart jar and pour tea over. Refrigerate overnight. Serve the next day with a hibiscus blossom floating on top!

DETOX!

You're a mess. You haven't been eating right — too many doughnuts and café mochas. You're not sleeping well, or you're trying to quit something. You've begun to notice that your body is waving a white flag. It's saying: "Help! Detox me and let's start over here." This section is a good place to start, as these teas are all excellent to support your proposed changes, body and soul. Today is the first day. Start now.

TURNING-THE-TIDE HAPPY CLEANSE TEA

2 parts burdock root

2 parts raw dandelion root

2 parts roasted dandelion root

2 parts sarsaparilla root

1 part echinacea root

1 part Oregon grape root

A classic blood purifier, this blend works through the liver and lymphatic channels. It's appropriate for anyone who is coming off sugar, drugs, or alcohol. Drink 2 cups per day. You can also make a tincture of this blend in brandy.

1 Add approximately 1 ounce of herb blend to 1 quart of boiling water, reduce heat, and simmer in a covered pot for 30 minutes.

2 Turn off the heat, and steep 30 minutes.

EMOTIONAL SUPPORT TEA

In addition to the previous recipe for the physical detox support, it's important to support the emotional side of detoxing. When addictions are addressed and positive dietary and lifestyle changes are being made, it's good to support the nerves and spirit too. Drink 2 to 4 cups daily. This is another excellent candidate for tincturing, so check out the section on making tinctures in the brewing chapter, pages 10–11. If alcohol is an issue, tinctures may be made in glycerin. If not, this is good tinctured in brandy.

3 parts St.-John's-wort flowers

2 parts chamomile flowers

2 parts oatstraw

1 part passiflora leaves

1 part red clover blossoms

1 part valerian root

⅛ part lavender flowers (organic)

① Combine all herbs in a pot, and cover with boiling water. Stir well, cover, and steep 15 to 20 minutes.

② Sweeten lightly with honey, if desired.

3-IN-1 REBUILDING ENERGY TEA

The ginseng and rehmannia nourish the adrenals and kidneys, the oatstraw feeds the nervous system, and the hawthorn supports the heart, making this an excellent tonic when rebuilding in the post detox phase. Take 2 to 4 cups daily, several days a week over a period of several months.

2 parts Siberian ginseng root

1 part hawthorn berries

1 part oatstraw

1 part cooked rehmannia root

1 part nettle leaves

① Combine all ingredients, except the nettles, in boiling water, reduce heat, and simmer for 30 minutes in a covered pot.

② Turn off the heat, add the nettles, and steep, covered, 30 minutes.

THE SWEET SMELL OF SUCCESS
Mindy Green
Boulder, Colorado

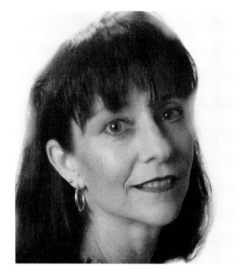

Mindy Green has made her varied living for the past 26 years in the herbal and natural foods marketplace. After a stint working in a health food store, she opened her own herb shop in Victoria, British Columbia. Other milestones on her herbal path include teaching at the California School of Herbal Studies and owning an herbal/essential oil company. She's a founding member of the American Herbalists Guild and currently holds the position of Director of Educational Services for the Herb Research Foundation. Over the years, Mindy's name has become practically synonymous with the word *aromatherapy,* and she's coauthored a book entitled *Aromatherapy: A Complete Guide to the Healing Art.*

Mindy knew as early as high school, after studying nutrition and realizing she could improve her own health through natural means, that her future was linked to the useful plants. She went on to receive a Master's degree in Health and Human Services and now writes magazine articles and books, teaches at the Rocky Mountain Center for Botanical Studies, and lectures in places far and near. She believes that sharing her experiences shows others a healthier way of life and gives them a sense of empowerment and cites the opportunity for continual learning and expanding her boundaries among the benefits of her work.

Her advice for the novice herbal enthusiast: Become familiar with simple herbal basics, learn to identify local medicinal herbs, and grow them in your garden. Mindy feels, for better or worse, that the future of herbs is headed toward mainstream consumption where quality may be compromised. "But there will always be the backyard herbalist," she says, "and my hope is that everyone gets some personal experience with that."

"Teas are the basic remedies of herbalists," Mindy says, "one of the best ways to know and understand the actions, appearance, and flavor of an herb." She also thinks the ritual of making and consuming tea is becoming a lost art. "Making tea takes time," Mindy says, "and people today are too busy and can't be bothered." She explains that taking a few minutes from a busy day to sit down with a cup of tea could significantly reduce stress in one's life. She recommends using the mild and flavorful herbs to introduce oneself or others to the pleasures of tea. "Many people are surprised herbs can taste so good," she says. Her personal pharmacopoeia always includes a variety of mints, nettles, and red clover.

MINDY'S MOVING EXPERIENCE

Mindy describes her favorite tea recipe as a bowel regulator (without the laxative effects of most bowel blends) and liver tonic (without the bitterness commonly associated with liver herbs), a good coffee substitute. "It has stimulating properties," she states, "a wonderful cold-weather beverage to keep you warm and nourished through the winter months."

3 parts burdock root

3 parts roasted dandelion root

2 parts raw dandelion root

2 parts roasted chicory root

1 part cardamom seeds

1 part cinnamon chips

1 part ginger root

1 part orange peel

1 part vitex berries

½ part licorice root

1 Add 1 to 2 teaspoons of dried herb mixture for each cup cold water in a pot. Bring to a boil and simmer, covered, 10 minutes.

2 Strain, sweeten with honey, and add milk (dairy or alternative) for more body.

A Seasonal Array

'Tis the season, whatever that season may be, because it's always the right season for tea, right? It's summer, for instance, and the living may or may not be easy, depending on how thirsty you are. But the cordial below will probably ensure your living *is* easy, or, trust me, at least easier. As a bonus, your garden is bursting with all the fresh herbs and flowers you'll need to further enhance these blends. Or, it's winter, brrrrrr, and there's 2 feet of snow on the ground. While you'll probably be relying on herbs of the dried variety for winter tea, they will still do the trick. We guarantee you'll enjoy the unique chai recipe that's included here, which is wonderfully spicy and warming, with no caffeine. Yum!

HIBISCUS COOLER SUN TEA

3 **parts hibiscus flowers**

2 **parts rose hips (organic)**

1 **part orange or tangerine slices (organic)**

1/10 **part cinnamon chips**

Honey or maple syrup (optional)

For a truly refreshing and deliciously unique beverage, add equal parts fresh apple and pineapple juice to this tea after it's brewed. If you are partial to a more lemony taste, add 1 part lemongrass or lemon verbena for some added zest.

1. Place all ingredients in an appropriate-size jar, cover with water, stir, and set in the sun for several hours.

2. Strain and sweeten with honey or maple syrup, if desired.

3. Serve iced.

ALL-SEASON CHAMOMILE CHAI

Chai is a traditional Indian spiced tea that warms the body and assists digestion. Most chai recipes call for some black tea, but this is made with chamomile instead, which makes it caffeine-free. This is delicious served hot before bed on a cold winter's night or blended with ice cubes and a scoop of vanilla ice cream on a hot summer's day! Vanilla soy milk, or honey and cream may also be added.

1 Combine all ingredients, except the chamomile, in boiling water, reduce heat, and simmer for 30 minutes in a covered pot.

2 Turn off the heat, add the chamomile, and steep, covered, 10 minutes.

3 **parts ginger root, freshly grated**

1 **part roasted coriander seeds***

¼ **part cinnamon chips***

⅛ **part cardamom pods***

1/16 **part whole allspice berries***

1 **part chamomile flowers**

Dry roast these ingredients together, stirring at medium heat until the coriander is golden brown.

SUMMERTIME & THE-LIVING-IS-EASY CORDIAL

Guaranteed to knock your socks off! All manner of unlikely amorous events have occurred after indulging in this brew: Hairstyles have spontaneously changed, women have become more beautiful, men have become more affectionate, and general merriment has ensued. You can add white wine or champagne, but you probably won't need to!

1 Rub the seeds of the angelica into a blender, add the fennel and water, and blend well, until the herbs are well liquefied.

2 Strain, discard herbs, and add the lemon or lime juice, with honey to taste. Serve chilled, in a pretty bowl with ice cubes and edible flowers (Johnny-jump-ups, calendula, rose petals, borage, and rose geranium work nicely).

1 **seed head fresh angelica (see caution on page 113)**

2-3 **cups freshly chopped fennel leaves, stalks, and flowers**

3-4 **cups water**

Juice of 2 or 3 lemons or limes (organic)

Honey, to taste

HERBAL ABILI-TEA
Brigitte Mars
Boulder, Colorado

"Drinking herb tea is a time-out in one's busy day for reflection and perhaps affirmation," says herbalist, writer, and teacher Brigitte Mars, owner of Uni-Tea Herb Tea Company in Boulder, Colorado.

Exposed early to herbal medicine at the knee of her French-Canadian grandmother, Brigitte, as a child, had her hair cut by moon phases and wore garlic medicine bags around her neck to repel colds.

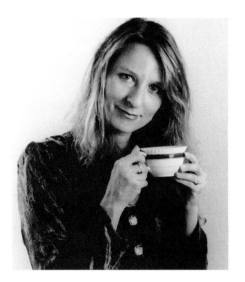

By the age of 15, she was trying herbal remedies on her classmates at school. Brigitte remembers that fellow students came to her rather than the school nurse. "It's my mission to help reconnect people with the power of the plant kingdom," she says.

In her late teens Brigitte moved to St. Croix, Virgin Islands, and spent her days harvesting seaweed and aloe vera. After moving to the Ozarks, she lived in a tepee for more than two years eating just wild edible plants, giving Brigitte an herbal education few of us can imagine. Her two daughters, Sunflower and Rainbeau, were home birthed and raised on natural medicines.

Brigitte also worked for 14 years at a large natural foods market as their herbalist and says that even after studying herbs for 30 years, she's sure she will be a student all her life. "I'm the eternal flower child," she smiles. She reminisces about a day in 1985 when, after drinking a tea of gotu kola before a business meeting, she created the Uni-Tea company, its name a symbol of harmony between all creation. Uni-Tea is composed of 12 blends with such great names as Sereni-Tea, Sensuali-Tea, Femini-Tea, and Digestabili-Tea that can be found in over 1,400 stores across the country.

Her favorite herbs: nettles, dandelion, and violet, because they grow everywhere and are so versatile in their uses. "People need to honor the common plants," she says. "I love for people to realize that some of the most useful plants are the common weeds outside their doors." She advises the beginning herbalist to "read everything, study with everyone, learn to identify herbs in your area, and try each plant by itself to become familiar with it." Brigitte has written several books, including *Natural First Aid* (Storey Books, 1999), *Elder,* and *Herbs for Hair, Skin & Nails.* She has also created a CD-ROM titled *Herbal Pharmacy.* She teaches at the Rocky Mountain Center for Botanical Studies, Boulder College of Massage, and the Naropa Institute. Check out Brigette's Website at http://www.indra.com/~brigitte/.

BRIGITTE'S BEST BRRRRR-BLAST

This is a good tea for the cold season, warming and spicy. "Have a toast to a great winter with someone you want to be warm with," Brigitte suggests.

2 parts roasted dandelion root

½ **part cinnamon bark**

½ **part dried ginger root**

½ **part (decorticated) cardamom pods***

½ **part star anise**

*Available at most health food stores.

1 Crush all the herbs in a mortar and pestle or mix briefly in a blender.

2 Add approximately 1 teaspoon of the herb mix to 1 cup water, then simmer at a low boil for 10 minutes.

3 Strain. Add honey and rice or soy milk to each cup and garnish with a sprinkle of nutmeg.

Great-Tasting Pleasures

Liver cleanses and blood-purifying teas aside, these blends are pure pleasure. While these fabulous beverages are included primarily because of their taste, they have secret benefits that will be working behind the scenes. The Ginger-Berry Cooler is my personal favorite. No, it's the Hibiscus Cooler Extraordinaire. No wait. It's definitely the Tahitian Rose Lemonade, which makes me think of a sunny, island paradise-kind of place, you know, with an umbrella stuck in my drink. Sigh. So many choices.

Tahitian Rose Lemonade

3 fresh lemons (organic)

1 quart water

Honey or maple syrup, to taste

1 teaspoon pure distilled rose water*

1 teaspoon pure distilled orange blossom water*

½ teaspoon vanilla extract

Available in health food stores, herb shops, or Greek and Mediterranean delis.

Invented by an eight-year-old, this is an amazing and exotic recipe! It's the most unusual and delicious lemonade you've ever tried, with delicate flavors sure to transport you to a faraway place. Serve this to someone you're wooing and see what happens!

1 Make the lemonade by squeezing the lemons into the water.

2 Strain out the seeds and sweeten lightly with honey.

3 Add the remaining ingredients.

4 Serve in a punch bowl over ice, garnished with fresh flowers, such as borage, Johnny-jump-ups, calendula petals, or bachelor's buttons.

GINGER-BERRY COOLER

You can make many new friends on a hot summer day with this yummy brew in tow, because they're sure to want some of this absolutely delicious, quite unusual refresher. Freeze a batch in a plastic 1-gallon water bottle and bring on a hike or picnic. Or lug it along for those long, hot days on the river, at the beach, or at afternoon concerts in the summer sun, and sip it throughout the day as it melts.

⅓ cup ginger root, freshly grated

Honey or maple syrup, to taste

1 quart blackberry or raspberry juice

1. Add the ginger to 1 quart boiling water, reduce heat, and simmer in a covered pot for 10 minutes.

2. Turn off the heat, and steep 10 minutes.

3. Strain and sweeten.

4. Add the fruit juice, stir well, and freeze until slushy.

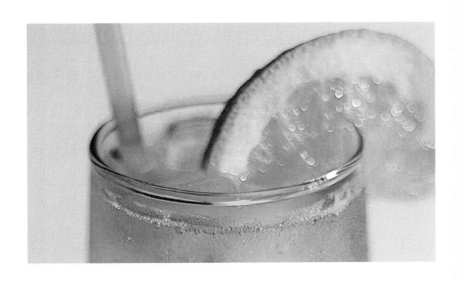

ICED LEMONGRASS-ADE

1 part lemongrass leaves

Honey or maple syrup, to taste

Lemongrass is a refreshing herb for summer, cooling to the body, high in vitamin A, and an all-around nice choice for a healthy iced tea. It's another good blend to freeze and take along on summertime outings.

1 Steep approximately 1 ounce lemongrass in 1 quart boiling water for 20 minutes in a covered pot.

2 Strain and sweeten lightly. Serve iced.

HIBISCUS COOLER EXTRAORDINAIRE

1 quart Hibiscus Cooler Sun Tea (see page 94), with sweetener omitted

3 cups apple juice (fresh is a must!)

1½ cups pineapple juice

This beverage turns a beautiful purple color from the acid reaction of the hibiscus and pineapple juice. It's absolutely delicious. Served hot or cold, it also freezes well. It's extremely thirst quenching for hot summer days. For postmarathons, long hikes, or other athletic endeavors, this is the best!

● Prepare the Hibiscus Cooler Sun Tea (you can omit the sun and just make a tea by usual methods), then add the fruit juices. Enjoy!

HOT BRANDIED-APPLE TODDIES

In addition to being a great winter warmer, this beverage is also wonderful for colds, coughs, hoarseness, and sore throats. Add a dollop of whipped cream per cup, if drinking just for fun!

1 Simmer all the ingredients, except the lemon, for 15 to 20 minutes in a covered pot.

2 Strain, and add fresh lemon juice and a shot of brandy.

2 cups apple juice

2 cups water

Fresh lemon and orange slices (organic)

1-2 cinnamon sticks

5-6 whole cloves

1-2 tablespoons ginger, freshly grated

Juice of 1 lemon

Brandy

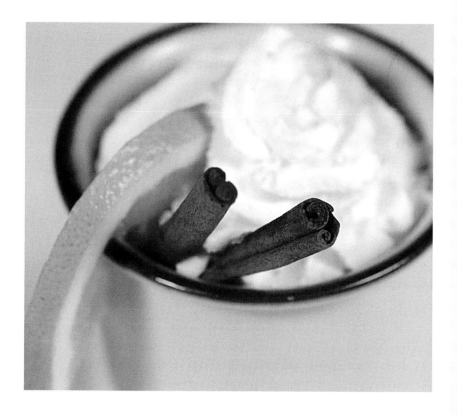

SOWING HER OATS
Suzanne Elliot
LaGranada, California

From one of her early experiences with herbs where she "learned the hard way," Suzanne Elliot remembers an incident where, as part of a gift basket for a couple, Suzanne made a bath scrubber bag for them to share. It was only after they laughingly confessed they itched all over from their bath that Suzanne realized the herbs "with hair on them" weren't the best for bath bags! From these inauspicious beginnings, Suzanne went on to create Wood-

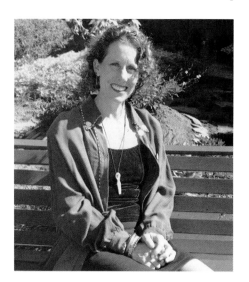

sorrel, a company that produces handmade herbal body and bath products, no doubt putting that early lesson to good use.

Suzanne first became interested in herbs over 20 years ago while working at a plant nursery. "I am compelled by herbs, they constantly speak to me," she says, counting tremendous benefits from working and communing with plants. Additionally, she is a shiatsu practitioner, has a consulting practice, and is an active teacher. She believes that people hunger for herbal knowledge and enjoys passing on her own information and experiences. She particularly credits Rosemary Gladstar, adding "I owe many of my formulating skills to her." In addition to her body products line, Suzanne has developed many herbal tea formulas, which she shares through her workshops.

"I love using herbal teas as therapy," she explains. "I believe it's important to taste what your medicine is about, and the process of preparing your medicine can be almost as important as what's inside."

Suzanne suggests to neophyte herbal tea drinkers that the taste and appearance are important factors in blending teas. "A medicine doesn't have to taste horrid to work," she adds. "It's important to challenge the taste buds because through the taste the whole organ system is affected." She also thinks it is important to present the teas in a visually pleasing way.

One of Suzanne's favorite herbs is oatstraw because it's simple, yet powerful, very nourishing, and gentle enough for children. One of her favorite rituals is gathering wild oats in the spring, stalk and all. She then cuts or bends four or five stalks into a quart pan of boiling water, covers, and steeps 15 to 20 minutes. After straining, she drinks this wonderful nerve tonic, high in calcium with a slightly sweet taste. She calls this her Gypsy Wild Oats Tea, and it is a pleasing sight indeed to picture Suzanne gathering her oats, then sowing them in her teas. "Continuing to learn more about herbs and using them for my own health have been truly empowering," she says.

SUZANNE'S SIMPLE SENSATION

This is Suzanne's favorite beverage, a lavish and lovely lemonade, both beautiful and refreshing.

2-3 handfuls fresh lavender or rose petals (organic) (half this amount, if dried)

1 cup fresh lemon juice (organic)

½–¾ cup honey or maple syrup

1. Pour 5 cups of boiling water over herbs in pan and cover. Steep 10 to 15 minutes.

2. Strain, then add the lemon juice and sweetener. Serve with floral ice cubes!

LOVE POTIONS

The candles are shimmering, there's some soft music playing in the background, and romance is in the air. After the gourmet dinner, you slip into something more comfortable — in this case, the kitchen — and return with, what else, a love potion. Serve it in a beautiful teapot and cups. Create mood from within. Give it a try. What have you got to lose?

CRIMSON LOVE TEA

2 **parts hibiscus flowers**

1 **part fennel (fresh leaves, stalks, flowers, and seeds, or dried seeds)**

1 **part rose hips (organic)**

½ **part star anise**

¼ **part rose petals (organic)**

¼ **part tangerine slices (organic)**

This potion has beautiful color and exotic flavor. Serve steaming hot on a chilly night, or it's great iced for romantic adventures in warmer weather.

1 Combine all herbs in a pot, and cover with boiling water.

2 Stir well, cover, and steep 15 to 20 minutes.

3 Serve with a little honey or maple syrup, if desired, as it's pretty "tangy" otherwise.

Aphrodisiac Honey — A Kissing Potion Extraordinaire!

Guaranteed by our recipe goddess to make a man propose! It's so simple, you'll be amazed at the results. To 2 ounces of honey, add 1 drop of pure rose geranium and lemon verbena essential oils. Stir well and let sit 1 hour at room temperature. This is delicious in tea, on toast or biscuits, or even applied to and licked from body parts of your choice!

DANCING DAMIANA DREAM

You'll be dancing cheek to cheek with that special person after drinking this potion. It's so tasty you may want to skip the dancing altogether. Ho, ho.

1. Combine all the herbs in a pot, and cover with boiling water.

2. Stir well, cover, and steep 15 to 20 minutes.

1 part chamomile flowers

1 part damiana leaves

1 part lemongrass leaves

1 part spearmint leaves

½ part passiflora leaves

¼ part jasmine flowers

¼ part orange peel/slices (organic)

PRETTY TEA

A visually gorgeous blend, this tea is aromatic and happiness enhancing! Not only is it great hot or iced and festive for holidays, it's good for digestion, too.

1. Combine all herbs in a pot, and cover with boiling water.

2. Stir well, cover, and steep 15 to 20 minutes.

1 part ginger root, freshly grated

1 part lemon verbena leaves

1 part peppermint or spearmint leaves

1 part rose hips (organic)

½ part orange slices (organic)

½ part rose petals (organic)

¼ part jasmine flowers

QUEEN OF JUICE
Diana De Luca
Sebastapol, California

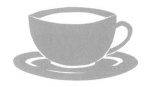

Diana De Luca, a colorful herbalist in Sonoma County, California since 1980, presents work and "play" shops throughout the United States and Canada on herbal folk ways, women's natural health care, belly dancing, and sensuality through herbs. My initial (and hopefully not last) encounter with Diana was at a seminar she taught at the Women's Herbal Conference on erotic herbs, where one of her favorite adjectives was

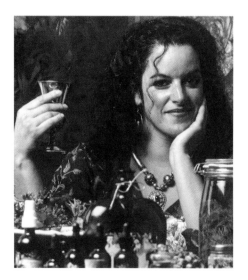

"juicy," giving new meaning to the word as applied to life, love and the pursuit of herbs! She mentions that one of her friends dubbed her "queen of juice," while another referred to her as "suca de luca," meaning "juice of light."

Diana learned about herbs and natural diet at her mother's knee, and credits both her mother and Rosemary Gladstar as her greatest inspiration for the herbal path she has followed ever since. "I grew up drinking red raspberry tea for PMS," she says. "We'd go into the foothills near Reno, Nevada to pick Mormon Tea." Diana fondly remembers sassafras tea with honey and lemon in the summer, and laughingly recalls going to school with "yellow fingers" as a child, from filling capsules with goldenseal.

Diana draws upon her rich Sicilian-American heritage and love of all things edible and aromatic to share her passion of green medicine in her products and her classes. She worked eight years as an herbalist for a natural food store, including three years for Rosemary's

Garden, and now has her own line of what she describes as "sensual herbal skin care," called Botanica Erotica. Diana brings this same exotic sensuality to her work as author of a book of the same name, *Botanica Erotica: Arousing Body, Mind, and Spirit.*

She likens her relationships with plants to her associations with friends. "I connect with the plants throughout the year and dance with the herbs inspired by each season," Diana explains. As for her thoughts about making herbal tea, Diana describes the time it takes to make your medicine, waiting for the kettle to boil, is the most important part of the process. "You have to sit still," she says.

PEACE ON EARTH

Diana recommends this blend for any time you need a supportive "attitude adjustment." It's good for stress, anxiety, PMS, or whatever's got you down.

1 Combine all the herbs in a jar and infuse.

2 Strain, and drink ½ to 1 cup as needed throughout the day.

3 parts skullcap leaves

2 parts passiflora leaves

1 part chamomile flowers and leaves

1 part spearmint leaves

Pinch of stevia

Sinful Blackberry Cordial

2 cups blackberries

1 handful ginger root, freshly grated

1 tablespoon cinnamon chips

2-3 thin orange slices (organic)

Honey

Go out to your favorite blackberry patch and gather lots. You'll want plenty of this cordial around. Take 1 to 2 tablespoons per day. Great over ice cream.

1. Gently crush the berries and place in a widemouthed jar with the rest of the ingredients.

2. Cover with three times as much brandy, and cap tightly.

3. Shake daily for several days, then strain. Sweeten lightly with honey.

4. Let it steep longer, if you can resist all urges to drink it! I've let some cordials sit for several years, and they turned out fantastic!

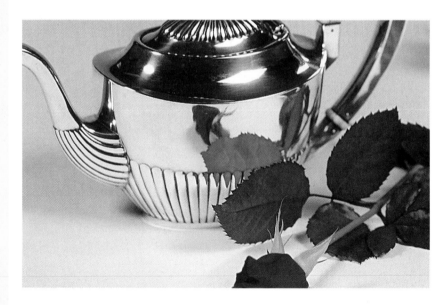

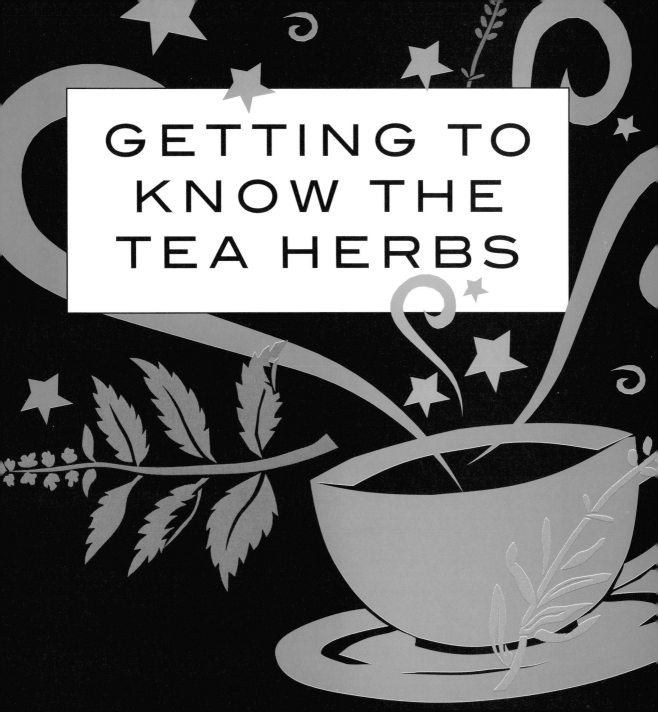

GETTING TO KNOW THE TEA HERBS

This chapter is offered to give you a quick reference to all of the herbs used in the recipes in this book. We haven't gone into depth, since this is not meant to be a comprehensive herb encyclopedia, but just given you enough information to get started on understanding the actions of each herb and how to use it in tea. We encourage you to explore the herbs in more depth with a comprehensive resource book (see Resource Books) or a class in herbalism taught by an experienced herbalist.

Following are definitions of some of the terminology commonly used by herbalists to describe the medicinal properties of herbs.

GLOSSARY OF MEDICINAL PROPERTIES

Alterative — produces gradual beneficial change in body, usually improvement through nutrition/metabolism. Examples: red clover, nettle, sarsaparilla, dandelion, yellow dock root, burdock root, alfalfa.

Anesthetic — deadens sensation, often contains salicin. Examples: rosemary, willow bark, poplar buds, kava-kava.

Anodyne — soothes or relieves pain. Examples: St.-John's-wort, valerian, wild poppy, calendula, plantain.

Anthelmintic — destroys or expels intestinal worms. Examples: wormwood, quassia chips, black walnut hulls, garlic.

Antiemetic — counteracts nausea and relieves vomiting. Examples: peppermint, chamomile, fennel.

Antiseptic — destroys or inhibits pathogenic or putrefactive bacteria. Examples: usnea, echinacea, sage, lemon, goldenseal.

Antispasmodic — relieves or checks spasms or cramps. Examples: St.-John's-wort, rosemary, chamomile, lavender.

Appetizer — excites the appetite. Examples: gentian, ginger, angelica, cardamom, fennel, Oregon grape root.

Aromatic — having an agreeable odor and stimulating qualities. Examples: mint, fennel, chamomile, lavender.

Astringent — contracts and lightens tissue, reducing secretions or discharges. Examples: black tea, chamomile, yarrow, lemon.

Carminitive — expels gas from the intestines. Examples: fennel, peppermint, cardamom, ginger, cinnamon, chamomile.

Carthartic — empties the bowels, laxative. Examples: senna, coffee berry, cascara sagrada.

Demulcent — soothes/protects/heals irritated tissue. Examples: plantain, chickweed, mullein, calendula.

Diaphoretic — promotes perspiration. Examples: elder, yarrow, peppermint, ginger.

Diuretic — increases the secretion and expulsion of urine. Examples: dandelion, nettle, parsley, burdock, chickweed.

Emetic — causes vomiting. Examples: lobelia, ipecac, goldenseal, salt water.

Emmenagogue — promotes menstrual flow. Examples: angelica, ginger, blue/black cohosh, pennyroyal, motherwort.

Emollient — used externally to soften and soothe. Examples: malva, calendula, borage, primrose, and violet flowers.

Expectorant — promotes discharge of mucus from respiratory passages. Examples: ginger, cayenne, yerba santa.

Febrifuge — reduces or eliminates fever. Examples: elder flower, yarrow, rosemary, lemon water.

Hemostat — stops bleeding. Examples: shepherd's purse, beth root, nettle, goldenseal, yarrow (external as well).

Nervine — having a calming or soothing effect on the nerves. Examples: valerian, wild oat, St.-John's-wort, chamomile.

Purgative — promotes vigorous emptying of the bowels. Examples: senna, coffee berry, cascara sagrada.

Sedative — soothing agent, reducing nervousness. Examples: wild lettuce, passiflora, valerian, chamomile, hops.

Stimulant — excites or quickens activity or physiological processes. Examples: yerba maté, guarana, green tea, mint.

Tonic — strengthens or invigorates organs or entire body. Examples: nettle, red clover, wild oat, burdock, dandelion.

health benefits:

- Stimulates appetite and aids in digestion, especially chronic and acute weaknesses
- Aids in assimilation of protein, carbohydrates, iron, and calcium
- Builds blood, regenerating normal strength and vitality
- Cools inflammatory symptoms associated with degeneration and aging

health benefits:

- Stimulates digestion
- Relieves flatulence
- Eases diarrhea and upset stomach
- Has stimulant and antiseptic properties

ALFALFA *(Medicago sativa)*

European herbalists knew about the soothing and strengthening qualities of alfalfa centuries ago, but it wasn't brought to the United States until 1850. Alfalfa is one of the few plants that heals the soil in which it grows, with roots as deep as 68 feet that break up heavy clay and bring up valuable nutrients from the subsoil. It is a rich source of fourteen of the sixteen principal mineral elements, such as calcium, iron, phosphorus, potassium, and magnesium, as well as essential enzymes. Alfalfa also contains vitamins A, D, E, G, K, and P. Legend has it that a house in which alfalfa grows will never want, as it is an herb of providence.

Part used for tea: Leaves
Taste: Grassy, pleasant, mild
How to brew: Infuse.

ALLSPICE *(Pimenta dioica)*

Grown mainly in Jamaica, the reddish-brown berries were introduced to Europe by Columbus who mistakenly thought it was pepper, hence its Spanish name *pimenta,* which means pepper. Although unripe, the berries are picked green because they lose their aroma as they ripen. The trees bear fruit after 6 to 7 years and can live 100 years or more. Allspice contains 4 percent volatile oil, plus proteins, lipids, minerals, and vitamins A, B, and C. Buy allspice whole and grind it as needed.

Part used for tea: Berries
Taste: Warm, spicy, aromatic
How to brew: Bruise berries in a mortar and pestle, then infuse.

ANGELICA *(Angelica archangelica* syn. *A. officinalis)*

Angelica is also known as St. Michael's plant, since it blooms on May 8 (his day). In the fifteenth and sixteenth centuries, herbalists thought a bag of angelica leaves tied around a child's neck would protect against witchcraft and evil spells. Formerly called *herba angelica* (angel's plant), it was reputed to have heavenly powers against disease. Legend has it that its name comes from a monk's dream where an angel revealed that this relative of parsley would cure plague.

Part used for tea: Seeds, leaves, and roots
Taste: Aromatic, bitter, maplelike flavor that slightly numbs the mouth
How to brew: Infuse leaves or crushed seeds or decoct roots.
Caution: Do not take during pregnancy. In large doses, it can have negative effects on blood pressure, heart action, and respiration. Also, don't confuse angelica with other umbelliferaes, such as water or poison hemlock and wild parsley, that look similar but are deadly poisonous!

health benefits:

* Relieves symptoms of colds, coughs, and bronchitis
* Soothes indigestion, flatulence, and colic
* Encourages menstruation
* Improves blood flow, useful in cases of poor circulation
* Seeds offer euphoric and diuretic actions
* Eases symptoms of exhaustion and sore muscles when added to the bath

ANISE *(Pimpinella anisum)*

Native to the Middle East, anise is one of the oldest known spices. It traveled with the Romans throughout Europe and England and was so popular in the Roman Empire that taxes were levied on it. In the sixteenth century, anise was widely used as mousetrap bait. One of the first herbs brought to America, where Shakers grew it as a medicinal crop, it is now used as a flavoring agent in candies and liqueurs. Caraway, cumin, dill, and fennel are close cousins. Placing an anise flower under your pillow is said to keep nightmares away.

Part used for tea: Seeds
Taste: Aromatic, sweet, licorice-like
How to brew: Bruise seeds in a mortar and pestle, then infuse.

health benefits:

* Eases symptoms of indigestion, nausea, flatulence, and colic
* Provides expectorant properties when added to cough medicines
* Helps relieve colic in infants
* Masks the taste of bitter herbs
* Promotes milk production in nursing mothers

- Purifies blood, neutralizing toxins
- Useful in treating skin conditions such as eczema, boils, acne, sores, and psoriasis
- Encourages elimination of uric acid via the kidneys
- Stimulates the liver and digestive system
- Helps regulate blood sugar

BURDOCK *(Arctium lappa)*

Burdock is an ancient herb, arriving with the colonists and quickly escaping to become a hardy weed. It's high in iron and other important minerals, and roots contain 45 to 50 percent inulin, a plant starch that seems to have a favorable effect on the pancreas and spleen. Burdock is a well-known vegetable, also known as "gobo," used in soups, stir-fries, and sushi. Folklore says to place burdock leaves on wrists and ankles helps to drain away fever. Can you believe that burdock served as the inspiration for the ubiquitous Velcro? It's true — the Swiss inventor, George de Mestral, developed Velcro after observing the tiny hooks on burdock seeds.

Part used for tea: Root, collected in autumn or spring of second year. Fresh or dried.

Taste: Sweetish, slightly bitter, earthy

How to brew: Decoct freshly chopped or dried cut-and-sifted root.

health benefits:

- Stimulates digestion
- Relieves flatulence and eases bowel spasms and symptoms of stomach disorders
- Chewing the seeds sweetens the breath
- Eases the cramping effects of laxatives when combined with bitter remedies
- Improves the taste of bitter formulas, especially when combined with ginger and orange

CARDAMOM *(Elettaria cardamomum)*

Cardamom is the third most expensive spice (after saffron and vanilla) and one of the most ancient, called the "Queen of Spices" in India. It enhances both sweet and savory tastes. The flavor is in the small, hard seeds. Although the pod is inedible, Arabs put them in the spouts of their coffeepots to give the drink a distinctive taste, and in our recipes, the pods are included so they can release their flavor. Scandinavians are the largest importers, using it extensively for flavoring cakes, pastries, and bread. It is one of the main ingredients in garam masala and curry powder and, although its use has been primarily culinary, it is known to have medicinal value as well. Legend has it that to carry or consume cardamom is to draw love and passion into your life.

Part used for tea: Seeds

Taste: Initially a penetrating note of camphor, bitter and aromatic, then the taste lingers in the mouth in a warming and agreeable way.

How to brew: Bruise seeds in a mortar and pestle, then infuse. Use sparingly, as it has a strong flavor.

CATNIP *(Nepeta cataria)*

Besides being much beloved by cats everywhere, catnip was used by Romans as a tea and by people of the Middle Ages to flavor salads and meat. It was a commercial crop in colonial America. A first cousin to mint, catnip contains vitamin C and is renown for its relaxant properties. Legend says that two friends clasping fresh catnip between their hands will remain close forever. Placed around the home, this herb promotes improved fortunes.

Part used for tea: Leaves
Taste: Aromatic, minty, pungent, musty
How to brew: Infuse.
Caution: Catnip should not be used during pregnancy as it increases menstrual flow.

health benefits:

* Eases symptoms of flu, colds, and bronchitis
* Helps a restless child sleep
* Relieves the discomfort of stomach disorders, including colic, spasms, flatulence, and acidity
* Calming action for hysteria, nervousness, and headaches
* Cleanses and heals the lower bowel when used as an enema
* Externally, a tincture can be used as a friction rub for arthritis

CELERY *(Apium graveolens)*

What we know today as celery comes from a wild variety called *smallage*, used since ancient times as medicine. This bitter herb signified ill fortune and death and was used to make funeral wreaths, but in the seventeenth century, the bitterness was bred out and now all parts — stalks, leaves, seeds, and oil — are used for both culinary and medicinal purposes. It is a good mineral-rich cleanser, a diuretic herb, with detoxifying properties that improve circulation of blood to muscles and joints. A member of the parsley family, celery is said to improve prophetic ability and insight.

Part used for tea: Seeds
Taste: Warm, bitter, hint of nutmeg and parsley
How to brew: Bruise seeds in a mortar and pestle, then infuse.

health benefits:

* Reduces acidity in the blood
* Provides mild tranquilizing action
* Tones the liver
* Eases the symptoms of stomach disorders such as flatulence
* Promotes rest and sleep
* Offers antiseptic action for urinary problems
* Helps normalize blood pressure

health benefits:

- Soothes digestive disorders such as indigestion, diarrhea, cramps, and flatulence
- Offers moderate sedative and calming effects
- Relieves symptoms of colds and flu, especially when aches and pains are present
- Soothes irritated or sunburned skin or sore muscles when added to the bath
- An excellent hair rinse for blonds

CHAMOMILE, ROMAN

(Anthemis nobilis) and Chamomile, German *(Matricaria recutita)*

Known as the emblem of sweetness and humility, the name comes from the Greek words *kamai,* meaning "on the ground," and *melon,* meaning "apple," or "ground apple," as, when bruised or walked on, chamomile produces a delightful, applelike odor. Ancient Egyptians believed that it prevented aging, and in the Middle Ages, it was used as a strewing herb for its disinfectant properties. In monastery gardens, it was called the "doctor for plants," as it seemed to invigorate sick plants and promote healthy growth of all nearby plants. It's said that to carry a sprig of this herb is to attract money or love.

Part used for tea: Flowers
Taste: Light, applelike, slightly bitter
How to brew: Infuse.
Caution: The pollen in the flower heads is the same as in ragweed, so if you're allergic to ragweed, avoid this herb.

health benefits:

- Relieves digestive problems such as nausea and diarrhea, and strengthens weak digestion
- Eases the symptoms of colds and flu
- Stimulates circulation
- Offers antiseptic, antibacterial, and antifungal action
- Provides antiviral properties for aching muscles
- Stimulates the uterus and encourages menstrual bleeding

CINNAMON *(Cinnamomum zeylanicum)*

Native to Sri Lanka, cinnamon is one of the oldest herbal medicines and one of the first spices sought in fifteenth- and sixteenth-century explorations. Ancient Hebrews and Arabs used it as a perfume spice, placing a value on it equaled only by gold and frankincense. Egyptians used it for embalming, and, though known primarily for its culinary value in flavoring everything from meat to desserts, it has medicinal value as well.

Part used for tea: Ground bark and chips
Taste: Well defined, fragrant, sweet, spicy and warm
How to brew: Infuse.
Caution: Do not use during pregnancy as it stimulates the uterus.

CORIANDER *(Coriandrum sativum)*

Coriander seeds were found in ancient Egyptian tombs and have been used for more than three thousand years. This herb gained popularity when ancient Hebrews favored it as one of the bitter herbs of Passover rituals. Used today more as a spice than a medicine, it nonetheless has been used historically to treat a wide variety of maladies. Today, it's known primarily as a digestive tonic with mild antispasmodic properties. Used in both savory and sweet dishes, it is an essential ingredient in curry. Legend has it that a pregnant woman eating coriander ensures her future child's inventiveness.

Part used for tea: Seeds
Taste: Spicy, warming, a peppery-balsamic note, mild
How to brew: Bruise seeds in a mortar and pestle, then infuse or decoct.

health benefits:

❋ Soothes upset stomachs, promotes digestion, stimulates appetite, reduces flatulence, and aids in secretion of gastric juices

❋ Improves the flavor of other medicinal teas

❋ Rumored to have aphrodisiac effects

❋ Chew the seeds to sweeten breath

CRAMPBARK *(Viburnum opulus)*

Also known as Guelder Rose, cranberry bush, or "snowball tree" because of its round, white flower clusters, crampbark is native to both North America and Europe. It is grown ornamentally in the United States, where it sometimes escapes from cultivation. It remained in *The U.S. Pharmacopoeia* from 1882 to 1926 and was recognized as recently as 1960 as a sedative for nervous conditions and as an antispasmodic. Originally a Native American remedy, the bark is collected in spring and summer when the plant is in flower, and it can be used either topically or internally to relieve any cramping or tight muscles of intestines, lungs, uterus, limbs or back. In Russia, the berries are made into a brandy that they use as a peptic ulcer remedy, the Japanese make a vinegar extract to treat cirrhosis of the liver, and the Chinese use it as a laxative.

Part used for tea: Stem bark
Taste: Aromatic, bitter, woody, astringent
How to brew: Decoct.
Caution: The fresh berries are poisonous.

health benefits:

❋ Eases cramping during menses

❋ Helps prevent excessive uterine bleeding in menopause

❋ Relieves constipation, colic, and digestive cramping

❋ Tones and relaxes nervous system

- Useful in treating premature ejaculation and impotence in men
- Strengthens a woman's ovaries and eases menstrual-related headaches
- Provides diuretic properties and is slightly antiseptic to the urinary tract
- Offers tonic action for debility, depression, and lethargy

health benefits:

- Stimulates liver and gallbladder activity
- Benefits stomach and intestines, helping assimilate nutrients from food
- Eases chronic sluggish bowel
- Cleanses the blood, especially useful in treating congestive skin problems
- Leaves have diuretic properties, with high levels of potassium.

DAMIANA *(Turnera diffusa var. T. aphrodisiaca)*

Damiana has been used for centuries to enhance sexual prowess and balance hormones, traditionally an aphrodisiac of the Mayan people. A unisex herb and general tonic containing thymol, with strong antiseptic properties, it is life enhancing for both body and mind. Considered a tonic and stimulant, damiana has no caffeine. It offers especially good results in herbal formulas that address anxiety and depression after long-term stress. Damiana is best combined with other herbs that strengthen the nerves, such as oatstraw, rosemary, and St.-John's-wort.

Part used for tea: Leaves
Taste: Aromatic, slightly bitter
How to brew: Infuse.
Caution: Damiana should not be used continually as it interferes with iron absorption and too much of this herb may cause insomnia and headache and irritate the bladder.

DANDELION *(Taraxacum officinale)*

Considered a weed by farmers and most gardeners, dandelion is found throughout the Northern Hemisphere and has an astonishing range of health benefits. It makes an excellent wine, and the roasted roots are touted as a viable caffeine-free coffee substitute. Containing vitamins A, B, C, and D, dandelion is an excellent, mildly bitter "spring tonic," its leaves high in iron and potassium. Dandelion has a high inulin content that aids in regulating pancreatic function. This helpful root tones the liver, kidneys, pancreas, and blood and has a gentle laxative action. The French call dandelion *piss en lit,* roughly translated as "piss in the night" or "piss in the bed," because of its strong diuretic properties. Dandelion is also believed to increase psychic powers.

Part used for tea: Leaves and root
Taste: Leaves: grassy, robust, bitter. Root: bitter, with a coffeelike taste when roasted.
How to brew: Infuse leaves. When using fresh root, chop and decoct. Decoct the cut-and-sifted dried root.

DONG QUAI *(Angelica sinensis)*

A unisex herb that stimulates both ovarian and testicular hormones, it is best known in Asia as the "female ginseng." According to lore, drinking dong quai tea delays aging in women, and it is taken by millions of women around the world as an invigorating tonic. It contains vitamin B_{12} and has both antibiotic and antispasmodic properties. The translated name of dong quai means "state of return," because it helps bring balance and harmony to the female cycle by building the blood and regulating hormones.

Part used for tea: Root
Taste: Bitter and aromatic, maplelike and smoky
How to brew: Decoct whole root.
Caution: Be aware that taking dong quai just prior to menses can cause a heavier flow, and don't take it during pregnancy as it's too stimulating to the uterus. Women using dong quai as a tonic should take it during the PMS phase each month or after menses for one to two weeks.

health benefits:

* Beneficial in the treatment of irregular menstruation

* Eases menopausal symptoms such as vaginal dryness, hot flashes, and emotional imbalance

* Increases circulation, nourishing to blood, and useful in treating anemia

* Soothes and calms the central nervous system

* Moistens the intestines to ease constipation

ECHINACEA *(Echinacea angustifolia* and *E. purpurea)*

Native Americans used this strong medicine for snakebite and as a pain reliever and antiseptic long before the colonists arrived. In addition, it was used in offerings to invoke support of spirits for magical works. It was the most popular plant in the 1920s, now cited as one of the world's most important medicinal herbs. Echinacea is known primarily as a powerful immune system stimulant and as a wonder herb that increases production of white blood cells to fight viral and bacterial infections.

Part used for tea: Root, harvested from at least three-year-old plants
Taste: Sweetish, woody, then pungent with a tingling sensation
How to brew: Decoct freshly chopped or dried root.
Caution: Don't take echinacea constantly — just when needed, when you're starting to feel ill. An echinacea tincture is particularly effective as a preventive measure during cold and flu season or if you have to be in contact with sick people or exposed to circulating germs in an airplane when traveling.

health benefits:

* Useful in fighting off colds and flu, especially at the onset of symptoms

* Purifies blood and lymph, useful in conditions such as eczema, acne, and boils that indicate impurities in the blood

* Aids in proper digestion by stimulating liver and digestive enzymes

* Chewing the root can ease discomfort from a sore throat or toothache.

health benefits:

* Dispels first-stage symptoms of colds and flu with antiviral action

* Externally, use as an antiseptic wash for skin problems, wounds, and inflammations. Used in salves for burns, rashes, and minor skin ailments and to diminish wrinkles.

* Promotes perspiration and urine production to remove waste products, of value in arthritic conditions

* Eases symptoms of digestive disorders such as diarrhea and flatulence

health benefits:

* Useful in herbal formulas for treating asthma, bronchitis, allergies, sinus problems, even the common cold

* Helps suppress appetite and stimulate metabolism, similar to caffeine

* Provides mild diuretic properties

* Reduces fever

ELDER *(Sambucus nigra)*

Elder has more folklore associated with it than any other European plant. Undertakers once carried pieces of elder to protect them against the numerous spirits they might encounter in the course of their work. Men doffed their hats in the tree's presence and offered prayers to the elder "mother" before gathering her berries, and Christians believed elder to be the wood of the Cross. It was once thought that to burn elder wood would cause one to see the devil, and it is believed that Judas hanged himself from the elder tree. Lore says to never use elder wood in cradle construction lest the fairies gain access to the child within. High in vitamin C, elder berries are popular for making wine as well as for their medicinal value.

Part used for tea: Flowers and cooked or dried berries

Taste: Flowers: sweet and honey flavored. Berries: tart, like blueberries

How to brew: Infuse.

Caution: The roots, stems, and leaves can cause poisoning, although the ripe, cooked berries and flowers are not considered toxic. Be very careful to use only blue elder flowers and berries, as the red elder is poisonous and very toxic.

EPHEDRA *(Ephedra sinica, E. intermedia, E. equisetina)*

Also known as Mormon Tea (American species) and *ma huang* (Chinese species), ephedra has been used for thousands of years in Chinese medicine as a powerful decongestant and bronchodilator. Its primary alkaloid, ephedrine, has been put to extensive use in both prescription and over-the-counter decongestants, and cold and allergy medications.

Part used for tea: Leaves and branches

Taste: Pleasant, pinelike, woody, slightly earthy

How to brew: Infuse.

Caution: Ephedra is a stimulant that can increase blood pressure and heart rate and cause insomnia and anxiety. People with thyroid disease, glaucoma, diabetes, enlarged prostate, high blood pressure, and heart disease or those using MAO inhibitor–type antidepressants should not use this herb.

FENNEL *(Foeniculum vulgare)*

Ancient Greeks consumed fennel to obtain courage and long life and to honor Adonis. Romans used it to keep a trim waistline. In the Middle Ages, it was considered one of several sacred herbs that cured disease. Fennel seeds are a symbol of heroism. Primarily a culinary herb, it has a long history of medicinal use and is known today as an excellent stomach and intestinal remedy. Fennel is great used in cold and cough tea formulas as it moistens and soothes the throat, and it's helpful in making a bitter tea more palatable.

Part used for tea: Seeds and fresh leaves, stalks, and flowers

Taste: A combination of anise and licorice, delightful, sweet and slightly bitter

How to brew: Bruise seeds in a mortar and pestle, then infuse.

Caution: If picking fennel in the wild, be sure you can distinguish fennel from other umbelliferaes, such as poison or water hemlock, that are highly poisonous.

health benefits:

* Arouses appetite
* Relieves flatulence, colic, and abdominal cramps
* Helps expel mucus accumulations
* Seeds boiled in barley water stimulate lactation in nursing mothers
* Soothes coughs and throat and lung
* Externally, use as an eyewash

FENUGREEK *(Trigonella foenum-graecum)*

Fenugreek is one of the oldest known medicinal plants, dating back to the ancient Egyptians and Greeks. Arabs use the roasted seeds as a coffee substitute, and it's known both as cattle fodder and as a crop that restores nitrogen to the soil. Fenugreek contains vitamins A, B, and C, calcium, iron, and steroidal saponins, which closely resemble the body's own sex hormones. Useful as a culinary flavoring, it has a maplelike odor and is a principal ingredient in curry. Fenugreek has medicinal value in reproductive and hormonal tonics and also provides soothing, mucilaginous actions for throat, lungs, stomach, and bladder.

Part used for tea: Seeds

Taste: Pleasant, bitter, reminiscent of maple and vanilla, a slight celery taste

How to brew: Quick-simmer 3 to 5 minutes. Fenugreek gets bitter if simmered too long.

Caution: Fenugreek should not be used during pregnancy as it has a stimulating effect on the uterus.

health benefits:

* Soothes lung and throat irritations
* Strengthens those recovering from an illness, especially for bronchial conditions
* Nourishes the endocrine system for hormonal balance
* Tones the liver
* Cleansing for blood and bowels

health benefits:

- Helps relieve symptoms of coughs and lung and chest problems
- Eases digestive problems, especially constipation
- Soothes, protects, and flushes the urinary tract
- Oil is useful in lubricating intestines and gallbladder

health benefits:

- Fights colds, coughs, and flu with strong antiviral and antibacterial action
- Helps lower blood pressure and cholesterol levels and to cleanse arteries
- Useful in regulating pancreatic function
- Externally, use oil for aches, sprains, and minor skin disorders.
- Stimulates digestion
- Aids in regulating liver and gallbladder action

FLAX *(Linum usitatissimum)*

Cultivated since at least 5000 B.C., flax contains valuable anti-inflammatory essential fatty acids. Both soothing and mucilaginous, it is helpful in a variety of conditions. Flax oil is popular as a tonic for helping balance the hormones and ease PMS. Eating 2 tablespoons of flax each day, freshly ground in a coffee grinder, can provide the essential fatty acids needed for a healthy heart, skin, and reproductive system. Sprinkle it on oatmeal or granola, or mix it into your morning smoothie!

Part used for tea: Seeds
Taste: Bland and nutty
How to brew: Steep or quick-simmer 5 to 10 minutes

GARLIC *(Allium sativum)*

Medicinally, garlic has been used as early as 3000 B.C. Ancient Egyptians swore on a clove of garlic when they took a solemn oath and ate garlic for strength, speed, and endurance as they built the pyramids. Once thought to possess magical powers against vampires and evil, garlic has historically been used in charms and spells. A world-renowned cure-all, it contains sulfur-rich compounds and allicin, which has strong antibiotic action, as well as vitamins A and B, fats, and amino acids. Known as "Russian penicillin," it was applied to wounds to prevent septic poisoning and gangrene in both world wars.

Part used for tea: Cloves
Taste: Warm and pungent, onion-y but much stronger
How to brew: Crush cloves, then infuse. Do not boil.

H'ear H'ear!

This is a good recipe for earaches. Infuse 4 crushed cloves of garlic in ¼ cup warm olive oil for 1 hour. Strain, then apply a few drops of oil in the ear or soak a cotton ball and place it in the ear.

GERANIUM, ROSE *(Pelargonium graveolens)*

The genus *Pelargonium* originated in the Cape of Good Hope in Africa and was introduced to Britain in 1632. The plants remained relatively unknown until 1847 when the French perfume industry realized their aromatic potential. In the summer, the Victorians lined their pathways with pelargoniums, where the women's long skirts brushed against the plants, scenting the air with their fragrance. In the winter, the potted plants were brought inside to release their fragrance into the rooms in the same way. In the Victorian language of flowers, geranium represents comfort and consolation, and it's reputed to protect a home from snakes.

Part used for tea: Fresh leaves and fresh or dried flowers
Taste: Depends on variety, each with its own taste. Rose geranium is rose flavored and citrus-y, with a hint of bitterness.
How to brew: Infuse.
Caution: Don't use sprayed plants for tea.

health benefits:

* Relaxes and tones the nervous system and lifts spirits
* Useful in baths and massage oils to relieve premenstrual tension and fluid retention through aromatherapy
* Eases the symptoms of dermatitis, eczema, herpes, and dry skin through aromatherapy and skin-care preparations
* Relieves dysentery, stomach disorders, and intestinal ulcers

GINGER *(Zingiber officinale)*

One of the most versatile herbal stimulants, ginger has been cultivated in Asia for more than three thousand years. In the Middle Ages, medicinal ginger beers were thought to thwart plague. During the 1700 and 1800s, it was one of the most popular culinary herbs throughout Europe. Ginger is extremely useful in relieving travel sickness and vertigo, proven to be as effective as Dramamine, without the drowsy side effect. Capsules, teas, even candied ginger works.

Part used for tea: Root, harvested 8 to 12 months after planting
Taste: Spicy, warming, aromatic, slightly biting
How to brew: Quick-simmer 5 to 10 minutes.
Caution: Some herbalists feel ginger is too warming and stimulating for use by pregnant women. Others use it in morning sickness formulas. Most of the ginger root available in markets is not organic, so be sure to scrape the skin off before using in the recipes; the edge of a teaspoon works well. Then grate or finely chop the peeled root.

health benefits:

* Relieves symptoms of cold, flu, and coughs, especially at the onset
* Helps relieve indigestion, cramps, vomiting, flatulence, and nausea
* Increases circulation, warms and increases vital energy
* Cleanses the colon and fights colitis and diverticulitis
* Eases symptoms of hangover and general debility

health benefits:

❀ Increases blood flow to the brain, easing symptoms of Alzheimer's disease, senility, memory loss, and depression

❀ Inhibits platelet activity factor to reduce blood clots

❀ Aids blood vessels in delivering oxygen throughout the body

❀ Reduces anxiety, tension headaches, and vision problems

health benefits:

❀ Improves the body's ability to cope with stress, both physical and emotional

❀ Increases immune function and resistance to infection

❀ Considered an aphrodisiac, strengthening both male and female reproductive organs

❀ Supports liver function

❀ Aids in digestion

❀ Helps regulate blood sugar and sustain energy

GINKGO *(Ginkgo biloba)*

Medicinal use of ginkgo can be traced back to Chinese herbals around 2800 B.C. where it was noted to "benefit the brain." The tree is the oldest on the planet, growing here for more than 200 million years. Ginkgo increases the rate at which information is transmitted at the nerve cell level, so it's widely used to treat age-related disorders. Rich in flavonoids, which strengthen the cardiovascular system, it's a great antioxidant for the whole body.

Part used for tea: Leaves, picked in September–October, just as they are beginning to turn yellow.

Taste: Sweet, bitter, astringent

How to brew: Infuse.

Caution: Do not exceed recommended dosages since it could lead to headaches or skin problems.

GINSENG

(Panax quinquefolius — includes Korean Red, Chinese Red, and Kirin)

For more than seven thousand years, the Chinese have valued ginseng root as a cure-all. It was brought to Europe in the ninth century and to the west in the eighteenth century. Used as a general tonic, curative, strength builder, aphrodisiac, and sexual rejuvenator, initially only the emperor and his household and favored friends were allowed to use this herb. The name comes from the Chinese word *ren shen,* meaning "man root," because the root resembles the human shape. It's one of the best tonics for blood, energy, and reproductive health, strengthening the basic cellular function of metabolism.

Part used for tea: Root, usually dug in autumn

Taste: Earthy, slightly sweet and bitter

How to brew: Decoct whole root, ideally in a double boiler, 2 to 3 hours.

Caution: People with hypertension should not take ginseng, and pregnant women should avoid it as it has too many hormonal constituents. Also, this is a tonic herb and should not be taken during colds, flu, or other acute illnesses.

GINSENG, SIBERIAN

(*Eleutherococcus senticosis*)

Siberian ginseng has many of the same properties as the *Panax* ginsengs but is considered less warming and safer for longer term use, with no tendency to raise blood pressure. This herb helps the body adapt to physical and emotional stress. It's been studied extensively in Russia, documented to enhance athletic endurance and mental clarity. Siberian ginseng supports the adrenal glands, which are responsible for many of our body's corticosteroids and responses to stress of all types. It's equally good for both men and women, supporting the entire endocrine system and helping nourish the immune and reproductive systems.

Part used for tea: Root
Taste: Bland, slightly sweet and woody, very pleasant
How to brew: Decoct either whole or dried cut-and-sifted root. It's usually sold as shavings of the root, but it's better to buy it as chunks or the whole root, if available.

health benefits:

* Enhances energy and vitality, particularly valuable as a tonic during times of stress and pressure

* Helps maintain good health rather than treat ill health

* Useful as remedy for exhaustion

GOLDENROD

(*Solidago odora, S. virgaurea* and spp.)

German settlers in Pennsylvania first made goldenrod into tea, then exported it to China. More than 80 species of goldenrod are found in the United States. The name comes from the Latin words *solidus* (whole) and *agere* (to perform), a testimonial to the healing power of the herb. Legend says that where goldenrod grew, buried treasure lay beneath. In addition, goldenrod appearing near your home might mean improved fortunes, and dowsers often used goldenrod stalks in their searches. With its antioxidant, diuretic, and astringent properties, it remains a valuable medicinal herb.

Part used for tea: Leaves and flowers
Taste: Bland, grassy, astringent
How to brew: Infuse.

health benefits:

* Soothes sore throats, reduces fever, stimulates perspiration

* Eases symptoms of urinary infections

* Helps flush kidney and bladder stones

* Acts against candida fungi; useful as douche

* Relieves chronic nasal congestion

* Useful as mouthwash and douche

- ❋ Stimulates the nervous system
- ❋ Offers anti-inflammatory properties
- ❋ Addresses urinary tract infections with mild diuretic action
- ❋ Tones and strengthens reproductive function
- ❋ Eliminates or counter-acts formation of mucus

health benefits:

- ❋ Helps normalize and regulate heart function
- ❋ Aids in lowering choles-terol levels, over time
- ❋ Balances and normalizes blood pressure levels
- ❋ Increases oxygen to the heart, working well in combination with ginkgo

GOTU KOLA *(Centella asiatica)*

Gotu kola has been an important part of Ayurvedic medicine in India for thousands of years, and in China it's known as a miracle elixir of life. An excellent blood purifier, it is used in India to treat leprosy. It is considered food for the brain, helping combat stress and depression, fighting senility, and improving reflexes, and works well in combination with ginkgo and Siberian ginseng.

Part used for tea: All aerial parts
Taste: Bittersweet, acrid
How to brew: Infuse.

HAWTHORN
(Crataegus oxyacantha and *C. monogyna)*

Known in the Middle Ages as a symbol of hope and "food for the heart," hawthorn is regarded today as a powerful heart tonic, relaxant, and antioxidant. Bioflavonoids present in hawthorn relax and dilate the arteries, especially coronary arteries, allowing more blood flow to and from the heart and reducing the degeneration of blood vessels. Early settlers used the tea to relieve kidney ailments and nervous conditions, including insomnia, giddiness, and stress. The Greeks called it *kratos,* meaning "strength," and the Chinese believe the heart is the home of the "shen," or spirit. When the shen is restless or disturbed, it may wander in the night, causing insomnia. Hawthorn nurtures and calms the heart, so the shen is able to come home and rest, thus allowing peaceful sleep.

Part used for tea: Flowers, leaves, and berries
Taste: Flowers are sweet scented and pleasant. Berries are bland and fruity, similar to crab apple. Leaves taste pleasant, a little like green tea.
How to brew: Infuse flowers, leaves, and crushed berries.

HIBISCUS *(Hibiscus sabdariffa)*

There are more than two hundred species of hibiscus, mostly the "garden" variety. The species used for tea is the genus given above, not usually grown in the United States. Hibiscus is rich in vitamins A and C and beta-carotene, making it a good antioxidant. Its organic plant acids and electrolytes content make hibiscus a great drink, either hot or cold, for athletes. Credited with aphrodisiac powers, hibiscus adds real drama to teas, fruit punches, lemonade, and beverages of all kinds with its bright, ruby-red color.

Part used for tea: Flowers
Taste: Very tart and lemony
How to brew: Infuse.
Caution: Be sure you are using the correct type of hibiscus for your tea making, as there are many types of ornamental hibiscus that do not have the correct flavor.

health benefits:

* Replaces electrolytes and quenches thirst during and after athletic endeavors
* Eases symptoms of colds, flus, and coughs
* Adds flavor and color to other blends

HOPS *(Humulus lupulus)*

Hops have been used since the fourteenth century, chiefly to brew beer. Romans ate young hop shoots like asparagus. Historically, the narcotic qualities of hops were considered a cure for uncontrolled sexual desires, especially as an antiaphrodisiac in men. In the Victorian language of flowers, hops signify injustice, and legend says hops bring sweet dreams and rejuvenation.

Part used for tea: Female flowers and leaves
Taste: Pungent, toasty, very bitter
How to brew: Infuse. Mix with some of the better-tasting herbs, such as spearmint and fennel, for added digestive benefit and to make the bitterness of hops more palatable.
Caution: Pollen from hops flowers may cause contact dermatitis. It is also not recommended for depressive illnesses.

health benefits:

* A strong nervine, encourages sleep by relaxing the nerves and calming the mind
* Useful in transition from alcohol, coffee, sugar, and the like, by calming and toning mind and spirit
* Stimulates appetite and relieves digestive disorders such as nervous diarrhea, flatulence, and intestinal cramps
* Addresses nervous irritability and a quarrelsome nature

health benefits:

❀ Contains easily absorbed calcium and silica

❀ Improves strength and elasticity of damaged or weak connective tissue

❀ Helps staunch wounds and nosebleeds, an excellent clotting agent

❀ Strengthens nails, teeth, and hair

❀ Externally, use in the bath to benefit sprains, fractures, and eczema.

HORSETAIL *(Equisetum arvense)*

With up to 40 percent silica content and high in calcium as well, mineral-rich horsetail helps support regeneration of connective tissue and mend broken bones. It has diuretic and astringent benefits for the urinary system, working well in formulas with other herbs for soothing and flushing the bladder. It's also useful in PMS and menopausal formulas for its mineral content and nourishing effect on the bones, joints, and hair. Known as "scouring rush," horsetail has a long history of being used to scrub out pots and pans along the banks of streams and rivers.

Parts used for tea: Aerial parts

Taste: Bland, pleasant, grassy

How to brew: Infuse.

Caution: Don't use horsetail for more than six weeks, as it may cause irritation of the digestive tract. Only use young spring horsetail, as it can concentrate any potential contaminants from the soil and water as it gets older.

health benefits:

❀ Soothes dry or sensitive skin, used in facial-care, bath, and massage products

❀ Oil is used in aromatherapy for its pleasant, exotic, elegant floral scent.

❀ Nourishes and softens mature or sun-damaged skin

❀ Relieves tension, a calming sedative

JASMINE *(Jasminum officinale)*

Introduced to Europe in the sixteenth century, jasmine was traditionally used in Buddhist rituals. Many think the scent of jasmine arouses erotic interests, and drops of jasmine oil massaged on the body were believed to overcome frigidity. Today jasmine is used extensively in the perfume industry and also used in both black and herbal tea blends for its delicate floral flavor. It's said that to wear jasmine perfume is to attract spiritual versus physical love. In the Victorian language of flowers, white jasmine flowers signify a friendly nature and yellow jasmine flowers represent poise and refinement. Carrying jasmine flowers reputedly attracts prosperity.

Part used for tea: Flowers

Taste: Fragrant and sweet, very heady, astringent

How to brew: Infuse.

KAVA-KAVA *(Piper methysticum)*

Used as a daily tonic, this herb has major ritual and cultural significance for the Polynesian people, who use it to communicate with their gods. Though the lactones in kava have a depressant effect on the central nervous system, it is also a tonic, making it a valuable remedy for a wide variety of disorders. Kava has a reputation as an aphrodisiac, providing both intoxicant and euphoric action, with analgesic, antiseptic, and diuretic properties as well.

Part used for tea: Root

Taste: Pungent, bitter, resinous, aromatic. Leaves mouth slightly numb.

How to brew: Quick-simmer whole root 5 to 10 minutes. Kava becomes too strong if simmered long.

Caution: Avoid prolonged use, as the resins in kava are hard on the kidneys. Regular use of large doses causes accumulation of toxins in the liver and can cause stupor, dermatitis, and yellowing of the teeth. Avoid kava during pregnancy. Also, while kava has been traditionally used for urinary tract infections and sexually transmitted diseases, we are not recommending it as a substitute for antibiotics.

health benefits:

* Eases insomnia, fatigue, and nervousness, giving a deep restful sleep with vivid, clear, and colorful dreams
* Cleanses and flushes the urinary tract
* Relaxes tense muscles, useful for chronic pain
* May benefit arthritic conditions with analgesic and diuretic effects

LAVENDER *(Lavandula officinalis* and spp.)

From the Latin word *lavare,* meaning "to wash," lavender is a symbol of tranquillity and purity. Ancient Greeks and Romans used lavender because of its clean scent and antiseptic/antibacterial properties, as a strewing herb and in their baths. It was traditionally used as a "smelling salt." Today, it is known worldwide for its volatile oil, used in perfumes, cosmetics, and aromatherapy.

Part used for tea: Flowers, picked when blossoms are at their prime

Taste: Sweetly aromatic, exotic flavor, slightly bitter, floral, delicate

How to brew: Infuse, using fresh or dried flowers.

Caution: Go lightly when using lavender in your tea blends. It can easily overpower the other herbs and make the whole blend too bitter. Be careful not to pick sprayed lavender. Grow your own or buy organic lavender.

health benefits:

* Helps relieve flatulence, nausea, and stomachaches
* Soothes, calms, and strengthens nerves, an excellent relaxant
* Eases muscle spasms and stimulates blood flow to muscles
* Relieves headache, migraine, dizziness, and fainting
* Masks unpleasant odors in houses, offices, and hospitals

health benefits:

❀ Dispels melancholy, lifts the spirits, reduces feelings of panic

❀ Relieves digestive disorders such as nausea, cramps, and flatulence, especially useful when overanxiety causes digestive problems

❀ Helps fight flu and colds

❀ Relaxes nerves and may relieve headache and migraine

health benefits:

❀ Used in treating digestive problems, relaxing stomach muscles, relieving cramps and flatulence

❀ Reduces fever, with an overall cooling effect on the body

❀ Externally, a gentle herb for facial steams and baths

LEMON BALM (*Melissa officinalis*)

Ancients believed lemon balm would ensure long life, and legend recommends it to bring joy. The name melissa is the Greek word for honeybee, who favor this plant. A member of the mint family, it is also known as "heart's delight" and "elixir of life." It is thought to renew youth, strengthen the brain, and relieve a languishing nature. Lemon balm is considered suitable for children. In the Victorian language of flowers, it represents social conversation, and folklore says it restores youth. Lemon balm is a mild and safe calming nervine, with anti-inflammatory and astringent properties from the high tannin content. It also contains antiviral compounds, which are useful in fighting colds, flu, and Herpes I and II.

Part used for tea: Fresh leaves are best, or freshly dried leaves
Taste: Lemony, refreshing, aromatic, cooling
How to brew: Infuse.

LEMONGRASS (*Cymbopogon citratus*)

Native to India and Sri Lanka, where it is known as "fever tea," this herb is primarily cultivated for its oil, used as both a culinary flavoring and as medicine. It has a delicious and mild flavor with refreshing and soothing properties, a wonderful addition to either iced or hot tea blends. Lemongrass mixes especially well with ginger or mints and can be extremely thirst quenching on a hot summer day. The oil contains up to 70 percent citral, which is antiseptic, and citronellal, which helps repel mosquitoes and bugs in external repellent blends. Also found in lemongrass are traces of essential oil components geraniol (found in rose geranium) and nerol (derived from orange blossom), which are relaxing and uplifting components used in skin-care products. Lemongrass is considered suitable for children.

Part used for tea: Leaves
Taste: Mild, lemony, fragrant and pleasant, grassy
How to brew: Infuse.
Caution: Do not use essential oil internally; avoid contact with eyes.

Lemon Verbena (*Aloysia triphylla*)

Native to South America, lemon verbena was historically used in finger bowls at banquets, and its oil is still used to scent soaps and cosmetics. It is also used for culinary purposes with fruit — in drinks, jellies, cakes, and homemade ice cream. Considered undervalued as medicine, lemon verbena has a delightful sweet lemon scent with calming and digestive effects. It has mildly antispetic, astringent, and anti-inflammatory properties and helps flavor other less-pleasant herbal blends.

Part used for tea: Leaves
Taste: Warm and lemony, clean and uplifting, very pleasant
How to brew: Infuse.
Caution: Long-term use of large amounts may cause stomach irritation.

health benefits:

* Tones and relaxes the nervous system, a gentle nervine and tonic
* Lifts spirits with tonic effect and aromatic scent
* Aids digestion and reduces cramps and nausea
* Soothes bronchial and nasal congestion

Licorice (*Glycyrrhiza glabra*)

The botanical name comes from the Greek words *glukus* (sweet) and *rhiza* (root). It is a commonly used herbal remedy. Chinese herbalists believe that licorice harmonizes, sweetens, and blends all the other herbs in a formula and also masks any medicinal taste. Chewing on licorice root has helped many people to stop smoking without gaining weight. Licorice contains glycyrrhizin, 50 times sweeter than sugar, with a similar structure to the hormones of the adrenal cortex, giving licorice its anti-inflammatory effect. Possibly, there are mild estrogenic effects as well, and it's been used traditionally in small amounts in reproductive tonic formulas.

Part used for tea: Root
Taste: Extremely sweet, like anise or fennel, with a slightly bitter aftertaste
How to brew: Quick-simmer 5 to 10 minutes, or steep.
Caution: Licorice should not be used by pregnant women, overweight people with edema, and those with high blood pressure or heart problems. Women with estrogenic-dependent breast cancer or a family history of breast cancer should avoid licorice. Using too much licorice can cause headache. It's a good support herb in other formulas but is not usually the basis of a blend, as it has serious potential side effects in large or constant doses.

health benefits:

* Relieves coughs, sore throats, mucus accumulation, and congestion
* Soothes digestive tract
* Supports adrenal function
* Strengthens and balances the female reproductive system

health benefits:

* Reduces tension and stress
* Relieves symptoms of colds, flu, and sore throats, reducing congestion and fever
* Soothes skin in facial toners with astringent properties
* Calms the mind and promotes sleep

health benefits:

* Relieves flatulence, cramps, nausea, heartburn, vomiting, and abdominal pain
* Helps ward off initial symptoms of cold and flu, induce sweating, and break fevers
* Eases headaches and other ailments attributed to nervous stomach
* Great flavoring for other herb blends

LINDEN (*Tilia* x *vulgaris, T.* x *europaea,* and spp.)

Lindens are among the most beautiful of trees, with their fragrant blossoms abuzz with honeybees. Historically, linden flowers have been used for a wide variety of remedies, ranging from keeping freckles and wrinkles at bay to stimulating hair growth. Also known as lime tree or basswood, linden has good calming properties, helpful in reducing stress and anxiety. Linden flower baths can calm irritable or restless children, and the flavonoid content improves circulation.

Part used for tea: Flowers, gathered when they smell strongly of honey

Taste: Warm, applelike, highly aromatic, astringent

How to brew: Infuse.

Caution: Linden is very astringent due to a high tannin content, so if you're drinking a large amount of linden tea, you might experience dryness in the mouth and throat. Be sure to drink lots of water (especially with lemon!) to rehydrate.

MINT, APPLE; PEPPERMINT; SPEARMINT
(*Mentha suaveolens, M.* x *piperita,* and *M. spicata*)

The mint species is characterized by its soothing, aromatic, refreshing, and distinctive odors and tastes, peppermint being one of the strongest flavors. The Chinese drink hot peppermint tea to cool off, as the diaphoretic properties open pores to let out excess heat. It contains menthol, thymol, and other volatile oils with antiseptic properties. Peppermint is the most widely used herb in the world, more stimulating to the circulation than spearmint and a stronger remedy for digestive problems. Apple mint, spearmint, and peppermint are all soothing to the digestive system and are considered safe for children.

Part used for tea: Leaves

Taste: Mints are aromatic and refreshing. Apple mint is delicately fruity, too.

How to brew: Infuse. Pour boiling water over fresh or dried leaves in a covered pan. Boiling mint not only destroys its volatile oil but ruins the taste as well.

MOTHERWORT (*Leonurus cardiaca*)

Motherwort's name translates as "the lion-hearted mother herb," a beautiful name for an herb so important that the Japanese have a Motherwort Festival on the ninth day of the ninth month, also known as "Month of Motherwort Flowers." With a long and colorful history dating back to early Greeks who gave this "mother's herb" to pregnant women, the flowers of motherwort are associated with long life. Besides its importance as a woman's herb, seventeenth century herbalist Nicholas Culpeper wrote that it would drive away melancholy vapors from the heart, and it is still known today as a valuable heart herb.

Part used for tea: All aerial parts
Taste: Very bitter and earthy
How to brew: Infuse.
Caution: The prickly leaves of motherwort can produce skin dermatitis when touched. Although traditionally given to pregnant women in the final stages of labor, this use is not currently recommended.

health benefits:
* Strengthens heart function
* Decreases muscle spasms such as menstrual cramps and heart palpitations
* Helpful in lowering blood pressure levels and slowing rapid heartbeat
* Reduces anxiety of childbirth, postpartum depression, and menopause
* Helps to lower fat levels in the blood

NETTLE (*Urtica dioica*)

Nettles are so rich in iron, protein, and vitamin content that it makes the effort of harvesting this nourishing and strengthening herb worthwhile. Known for its "sting," nettles are high in potassium and vitamins A and C, and nettles' iron content makes it a traditional treatment for anemia. With astringent and diuretic actions and high potassium content, it is a good choice in reducing symptoms of PMS and edema.

Part used for tea: Leaves
Taste: Bland, slightly tannic, robust, pleasant
How to brew: Infuse.
Caution: When handling or harvesting fresh nettle plants, which are covered with tiny stingers full of formic acid, be sure to wear gloves to prevent severe stinging, itching, and blistering where the plant touches the skin. Once cooked (approximately 10 minutes) or dried, nettles lose their stinging quality.

health benefits:
* Purifies, nourishes, and builds blood
* Builds adrenal and kidney function
* Nourishes core energy and helps deal with daily stress
* Strengthens pregnant women and increases milk supply for nursing mothers
* Helps moderate allergy response

- Calms, tones, and strengthens the entire nervous system
- Nourishes bones, teeth, hair, and cartilage
- Helpful in drug withdrawal, especially cigarettes
- Increases stamina and gently raises energy level

health benefits:

- Peel stimulates digestion and relieves flatulence.
- Inner peel and whole fruit useful in formulas for healing wounds, tissues, and bones
- Fruit is thirst quenching after exercise with vitamin C and electrolytes.
- Fruit improves waste elimination function.

OATSTRAW *(Avena sativa)*

Oats have a wide spectrum of value in human medicine. Containing B-complex vitamins, calcium, iron, copper, magnesium, and zinc, oatstraw increases strength of mind, body, and spirit. Formerly used to fill mattresses and well known to promote energy in horses (as well as humans!), oats have antidepressant, antispasmodic, and tonic properties. Legend says to carry a sprig to improve finances, and keeping a sprig in the home means everyone inside will never be hungry.

Part used for tea: Straw (fresh or dried stems) and spikelets

Taste: Delicate, pleasant, slightly sweet, and bland

How to brew: Infuse or decoct. Simmering 15 to 30 minutes helps draw out the minerals.

ORANGE *(Citrus sinensis)*

One of the most well known fruits in the world, most people are familiar with oranges for their culinary usage. But medicinally, orange has tonic and stimulant properties as well, providing a rich source of vitamin C that helps the immune system ward off infection. The inner peel (white part) is rich in bioflavonoids, which support vascular system health, and the bitter aspect of the outer peel stimulates the liver and digestive juices. Orange is particularly valuable as a flavoring in herbal mixtures, easing the bitterness of some remedies. In aromatherapy, orange blossom essential oil, called neroli, is very expensive and highly desired. Used in spells, orange peel promotes love and devotion. The Chinese believe that oranges draw prosperity. Tangerines, tangelos, or mandarin oranges can be used in any of the recipes instead of oranges.

Part used for tea: Flowers, fruit, peel

Taste: Sweet, juicy, citrus-y

How to brew: Infuse.

Caution: If taken in excess, orange can exacerbate arthritis, and those who are allergic to oranges should avoid this fruit. Be sure to use only organic citrus, especially when using the peels.

Oregon Grape

(Mahonia aquifolium syn. *Berberis aquilifolium)*

Ranked as one of the most outstanding Native American herbs, Oregon grape is high in the alkaloid berberine, one of the same active ingredients found in the endangered goldenseal plant, making it a viable alternative as an immune booster and antibacterial. It's also a good ingredient for bitter liver and digestive blends. Early settlers learned the value of Oregon grape from Indian medicine men, and its popularity boomed in the 1800s when it proved effective in treating infection. It was listed in official pharmacopoeias until 1950.

Part used for tea: Root, gathered after the second year in late autumn
Taste: Bitter, slightly astringent, cooling
How to brew: Decoct whole root.
Caution: Since it stimulates the liver, oregon grape should not be used by anyone with an overactive liver. Pregnant women should also avoid this herb, as it is too strong and bitter.

health benefits:

* Helpful in treating systemic infections with antiseptic, germicide, and antibiotic effects
* Stimulates liver activity and secretion of bile, strengthening weak liver function
* Purifies blood, making it useful for skin diseases such as psoriasis, eczema, acne, and cold sores
* Stimulates gallbladder, liver, and digestion

Parsley *(Petroselinum crispum)*

Early Greeks and Romans wore garlands of parsley at their banquets to absorb the fumes of wine and help prevent intoxication. Rich in chlorophyll, parsley was also eaten after dining to freshen the breath. Parsley is also rich in vitamins A, B, C, and K, calcium, phosphorus, thiamin, riboflavin, niacin, iron, and manganese. Cultivated all over the world, it is best known for its versatility in the kitchen. It nonetheless has valuable medicinal uses as a blood-building tonic. With vitamins A and C, beta-carotene, and iron, it's a good antioxidant, too. In the Victorian language of flowers, parsley represents feasting and entertainment, which is why it appears on restaurant plates so often.

Part used for tea: Leaves, harvested before the plant flowers
Taste: Refreshing, pungent, green, herbaceous!
How to brew: Infuse. Drink tea cool for best diuresis.
Caution: Pregnant women should avoid parsley, and very strong doses can be toxic or irritating to the kidneys and cause valuable minerals to be excreted.

health benefits:

* Nourishes reproductive system and tones uterine muscles
* Helps flush kidney and bladder, with good diuretic properties
* Stimulates appetite and strengthens digestion
* Externally, very soothing in skin lotions
* Chewing the raw leaf after meals can freshen breath

health benefits:
* Soothes and supports nerves
* Offers nonaddictive, mild sedative and tranquilizing properties
* Eases pain, tension, and nervous headache
* Helps decrease blood pressure
* Relieves PMS and menstrual cramps in combination with other antispasmodic herbs

PASSIONFLOWER (*Passiflora incarnata*)

Native Americans used passionflower long before the settlers arrived. It's not only incredibly beautiful to behold, a botanical jewel in the garden, it contains sedative alkaloids and flavonoids that are helpful in remedies for insomnia, restlessness, hysteria, anxiety, and hypertension. The name comes from the beautiful flowers thought to represent Christ's crucifixion — five stamens for the wounds, three styles for the nails, the flower's fringe for the crown of thorns, and the colors white and purple-blue for purity and heaven.

Part used for tea: Leaves

Taste: Bitter, cooling

How to brew: Infuse.

Caution: Some species of passiflora, both ornamental and wild, are toxic, so don't assume that all of them are useful. Use only the leaves of *Passiflora incarnata*, and don't exceed recommended dosages. In the recipes, we've referred to this herb as "passiflora leaves" to avoid confusion with passion flowers. It should not be taken during pregnancy, as it has too many alkaloids that could affect the fetus.

health benefits:
* Nourishes and purifies blood
* Relieves symptoms of cough, cold, asthma, and bronchitis
* Externally, useful in compresses and baths for rashes, ulcers, burns, and sores
* Supports nerves as relaxing and nutrient-rich tonic

RED CLOVER (*Trifolium pratense*)

Clover helps heal the earth as a regenerative mulch for depleted soil, replenishing nitrogen. It contains high amounts of protein and calcium and is a richly nourishing and purifying herb for the blood, traditionally used to help clear the skin. Clover is best known today as an excellent spring tonic. It gently nourishes, tones, and cleanses over time, often improving various metabolic functions. Traditionally, it has been used in herbal cancer treatment, and clover is also good in formulas that address the healing of bones, nerves, and muscles. It's also considered appropriate for healing use with children and was the favorite food for the mythical Brer Rabbit.

Part used for tea: Blossoms

Taste: Delicate, sweet, honey, floral

How to brew: Infuse.

Red Raspberry
(North American *[Rubus strigosus]* or European *[R. idaeus]*)

Raspberry has a long history in many cultures around the world as a pregnancy tonic. It has been given to pregnant women because fragarine, an active alkaloid found in the foliage, tones the female organs of reproduction, especially the muscles of the pelvic region and uterus. Raspberry is high in tannins with strong astringent properties and contains vitamins A, B, C, and E, pectin, calcium, magnesium, and phosphorus. It's cultivated for both culinary and medicinal purposes, and the wild variety *(R. strigosus)* is more potent than the cultivated variety *(R. idaeus),* which is most often sold commercially.

Part used for tea: Leaves
Taste: Robust, earthy, a little like green tea, tannic
How to brew: Infuse.
Caution: Because of their effect on the female reproductive system, raspberry leaves have acquired the reputation of being aphrodisiac and should be taken in moderation. The high tannin content can lead to constipation, especially in pregnancy, so serve tea with a splash of milk, soy milk, or cream to neutralize the tannins.

health benefits:
- Tones and strengthens uterine and pelvic muscles to encourage easy labor
- Eases diarrhea with astringent properties
- Externally, use as a gargle and a mouthwash for bleeding gums.

Redroot (*Ceanothus americanus, C. thyrsiflorus, C. cuneatus, C. integerrimus,* and spp.)

A member of the buckthorn family and close relative of *cascara sagrada,* there are more than 30 species of redroot in the Pacific Northwest alone. So named because the root has a rich, red color, it's also known as New Jersey Tea. It was one of the plants the colonists used for tea after they dumped the real thing in Boston Harbor. Redroot was used extensively by Native Americans for bowel complaints and swollen glands and is considered strongly antiseptic and astringent. It's excellent for lung and throat formulas when mixed with other herbs such as osha, echinacea, usnea, and ginger. Although it tastes much like China tea, it is currently not in favor as a tea substitute.

Part used for tea: Root bark of large root or whole root
Taste: Slightly sweet, woody, astringent, pleasant
How to brew: Decoct.

health benefits:
- Relieves swollen glands, tonsillitis, and mononucleosis
- Increases efficiency of waste transport from the lymph to the liver
- Cleans and tones liver, bowel, and spleen
- Externally, astringent properties make it a good gargle for sore throats

health benefits:

* Builds and nourishes blood
* Strengthens adrenals, kidneys, and liver
* Builds the body recovering from illness
* Relieves fatigue and overstressed nervous system
* Improves menstrual irregularity and infertility

REHMANNIA *(Rehmannia glutinosa)*

This herb is the cooked, prepared root of Chinese foxglove, an important Chinese longevity herb with deep nourishing action for the blood, kidneys, adrenals, and female reproductive system. The Chinese believe the kidneys are the seat of the "Life-Gate Fire" and to tonify the kidneys will ensure a long, healthy, and vital life. Mixing well with herbs such as dong quai and ginseng, it can be used for male and female tonic formulas.

Part used for tea: Cooked root

Taste: Smoky, sweet like maple syrup or dried apricots, pleasant

How to brew: Decoct whole cooked root.

What to Buy: Be sure to purchase the cooked rehmannia, called "Shu di Huang." The raw rehmannia, "Sheng di Huang," looks similar but is used in a completely different way.

health benefits:

* Hips strengthen heart and brain, rich in bioflavonoids
* Good for pre/post-surgery and healing from any structural injury
* Hips nourish blood and reproductive system
* Hips soothe sore throats and ward off colds
* Externally, the pure rose essential oil is soothing and uplifting to the nerves and spirit in baths, massage oils, and the like.

ROSE *(Rosa* spp.)

There are more than 10,000 rose varieties, the flower of love. Cultivated since the sixth century B.C., roses have been called "queen of flowers" and "gift of the angels." Rose hips are noted for their high concentrations of vitamins A, E, K, P, and especially C. A cup of rose hips is said to contain as much vitamin C as 150 oranges, and *Rosa rugosa* contains 3,000 milligrams of vitamin C per cup! Although the leaves aren't often used, the flowers are edible and are also used in all kinds of cosmetics, with aromatic and astringent properties appropriate for most skin types.

Part used for tea: Rose hips and petals

Taste: Hips are fruity, aromatic, sour, pleasant tasting. Petals are delicate, exotic, fragrant, like sipping a cupful of flowers.

How to brew: Infuse petals. Bruise hips in a mortar and pestle, then infuse.

Caution: Be sure to use only organic petals and hips, as they are often heavily sprayed. Do not take the essential oil of roses (or any essential oil!) internally without professional supervision.

ROSEMARY *(Rosmarinus officinalis)*

The symbol of friendship and remembrance, this evergreen shrub is said to bring luck and prevent witchcraft. Romans believed rosemary to be a symbol of fidelity between lovers. Placed under a pillow, rosemary is reputed to keep nightmares away. Early herbalists believed wearing a sprig of rosemary could cure nervous ailments and restore youth, and it was often burned in sick rooms to purify the air. Rosemary is a natural antioxidant and antiseptic and contains salicin, a natural painkiller and anti-inflammatory that is chemically similar to aspirin.

Part used for tea: Leaves and flowers
Taste: Piney and aromatic, resinous
How to brew: Infuse fresh or dried leaves and flowers.
Caution: Do not use the essential oil internally. Excessive amounts of rosemary can cause poisoning

health benefits:

- Stimulates circulation and brain function
- Eases joint pain and relieves headache
- Eases symptoms of indigestion, colic, nausea, and flatulence and aids in digestion of fat
- Promotes liver function and stimulates production of bile

SAGE (Garden *[Salvia officinalis]* and Black Sage *[S. mellifera]*)

There are more than seven hundred varieties of salvia, a member of the mint family. Its name comes from the Latin word *salare,* meaning "to cure," and it is indeed a valuable medicinal herb. Rich in a hydrocarbon known as salvene, sage has astringent, aromatic, stimulating, and bitter properties. Sage is thought to slow aging, enhance memory, and prevent hands from trembling and eyes from dimming. This is validated by an ancient Latin proverb that translates "How can a man die when sages grow in his garden?" It is considered estrogenic and tonic, and the volatile oil contains thujone, which is antiseptic but potentially dangerous (see Caution, below).

Part used for tea: Leaves and flowers
Taste: Aromatic, camphorlike, faintly bitter
How to brew: Infuse.
Caution: Large doses of sage, particularly the essential oil, can be toxic. People with epilepsy should avoid sage because of the thujone content, which can trigger epileptic attacks. Avoid sage tea if nursing, as it dries up breast milk.

health benefits:

- Calms and strengthens nerves, especially valuable in relieving nervous headache
- Cleanses, tones, and stimulates digestion and liver function
- Helps ease lung congestion; useful for colds and flus
- Externally, use to treat canker sores and sore gums, and as a gargle to soothe sore throats.
- Helps dry up milk in nursing mothers when ready to wean

health benefits:

- Relieves eruptive skin disorders such as acne, eczema, and psoriasis
- Tones the liver and purifies the blood
- Increases virility, potentially valuable in treating impotence and low libido
- Promotes healthy tissue growth for internal and external ulcers and wounds

health benefits:

- Purifies the blood and balances glandular function
- Eases symptoms of colds and flu
- Stimulates liver to remove toxins from system

SARSAPARILLA (*Smilax* spp.)

Historically, sarsaparilla was used by Native Americans to make a soothing, perspiration-inducing tea that was believed to alleviate rheumatism, gout, and skin diseases. It was used to treat syphilis from the sixteenth century to the discovery of antibiotics. Containing 1 to 3 percent steroidal saponins, this herb has traditionally been used to tone the glandular system and purify the blood. It is useful in endocrine-balancing formulas and is said to have aphrodisiac powers.

Part used for tea: Root, dug in autumn
Taste: Pleasant, woody, something like vanilla
How to brew: Decoct.

SASSAFRAS

(*Sassafras variifolium, S. officinale,* or *S. albidum*)

High in tannins, sassafras has astringent, cleansing, and purifying properties that are useful in treating skin problems. This member of the laurel family is also considered to have diuretic action, helpful in treating arthritis, gout, and rheumatism.

Part used for tea: Bark of the root
Taste: Root-beer flavor, spicy, warm, tannic
How to brew: Infuse bark or quick-simmer.
Caution: Tests on rats found that the major chemical constituent of the aromatic sassafras, safrole, is carcinogenic. Most herbalists agree that while safrole is especially strong in the essential oil, the oils in the plant are not very water soluble, so it is considered safe in small amounts for occasional use in tea blends. For instance, use 1/8 part of sassafras for every 1 part of other herbs. Never use the pure essential oil, and avoid during pregnancy due to possible danger to fetus.

SKULLCAP *(Scutellaria lateriflora)*

Skullcap was used by Native Americans long before it was adopted by European herbalists. Known to have excellent nervine, calmative, and antispasmodic properties, it is the herbal remedy of choice for all nervous disorders, including hysteria, convulsions, anxiety, stress, and insomnia. Once known as "mad dog weed," skullcap has been used to treat rabies. A member of the mint family, it is also said to soothe excessive sexual desires.

Part used for tea: All aerial parts

Taste: Bitter, drying

How to brew: Infuse.

Caution: Commercial dried skullcap is often adulterated with toxic herbs, so we recommend you (1) grow your own, (2) learn to identify and wildcraft it, or (3) buy a fresh tincture from a reputable source. Do not drink more than three half-cups of pure skullcap tea in any 24-hour period as excessive amounts can cause giddiness, stupor, confusion, and irregular pulse. It is safe in formulas with other herbs, particularly other relaxing herbs such as lemon balm and catnip.

health benefits:

* Tones, strengthens, and nourishes nerves
* Soothes nervous headaches, neuralgia, muscle spasms, and muscle cramps
* Strengthens and stimulates digestion, especially useful for nervous stomachs
* Great in PMS formulas to calm nerves and soothe the spirit

SQUAW VINE *(Mitchella repens)*

Historically, Native American women used this beautiful small trailing vine to hasten childbirth. With bright red berries in autumn, it's now commonly known as partridgeberry. It has also been called "twinberry" and "two-eyed berry," and was frequently used in Native American smoking mixtures. Containing saponins, alkaloids, mucilage, tannins, and glycosides, squaw vine is today a valuable herb for treating all types of women's disorders. In the early twentieth century, a tonifying and strengthening "Mother's Cordial" was made containing squaw vine, crampbark, blue cohosh, and unicorn root in a base of brandy. Squaw vine appeared in the *U.S. National Formulary* from 1926 to 1947 for uterine problems and is useful in promoting healthy hormone balance and fertility.

Part used for tea: Aerial parts and berries

Taste: Bitter

How to brew: Infuse.

health benefits:

* Aids labor and childbirth, with tonic action on uterus and ovaries, especially good when combined with nettles and red raspberry
* Normalizes menstruation and relieves heavy bleeding and painful menses
* Stimulates breast milk production
* Relieves fluid retention with diuretic properties

- Stimulates digestion and eases flatulence
- Moderates bitter flavor of most bitter digestive teas and tinctures
- Warming quality good for adding to winter cough/cold formulas
- Externally, chew to sweeten breath

health benefits:

- Strengthens and tones nerves and lifts the spirits
- Antiviral action against retroviruses such as herpes and HIV
- Useful in repairing nerve damage from trauma or injury
- Externally, fresh oil is soothing and promotes healing for scrapes, wounds, and burns

STAR ANISE *(Illicium verum)*

Native to southern China and Vietnam, this small evergreen tree, a member of the magnolia family, lives up to 100 years. The fruit has been used since the seventeenth century in fruit syrups and jams. It's been used primarily for culinary purposes in confections, gum, and liqueurs, particularly anisette. A commercial substitute for anise, its oil is used in soaps and perfumes, and it's frequently used to flavor medicines.

Part used for tea: Whole fruits

Taste: Similar to anise and fennel — pungent, licorice-like, with a sweet, spicy note

How to brew: Decoct whole fruits.

ST.-JOHN'S-WORT *(Hypericum perforatum)*

In medieval Europe, the flowers of St.-John's-wort were considered to have powerful magical powers that were put to use treating emotional and nervous complaints. Although it fell into disuse in the nineteenth century, it has once again become the herb of choice as an antidepressant, antispasmodic, sedative, and pain reliever. In 23 double-blind, placebo-controlled studies, St.-John's-wort proved 250 times more effective than the placebo for relieving mild to moderare depression, with few or no side effects. Although the flowers are originally yellow, they yield a beautiful red pigment when crushed and infused in oil or alcohol.

Part used for tea: Fresh or freshly dried flowering tops, picked in their prime (around the end of June)

Taste: Pleasant, earthy, lightly astringent

How to brew: Infuse.

Caution: Much of what's on the market is poor quality, with more stems and twigs than flowers, so look for the dried yellow flowers. Taking St.-John's-wort may cause photosensitivity, so take care if you're in the sun by applying sunscreen and/or appropriate clothing to cover your skin. Don't mix St.-John's-wort with other antidepressants unless under the supervision of your health-care provider.

THYME *(Thymus vulgaris)*

An early favorite of early Greeks and Romans, thyme was considered a strong antiseptic and credited with a multitude of powers, including antiaging. The ancient Egyptians used it as an embalming herb, and Europeans believed that eating thyme would allow one to glimpse fairies. Reputed to overcome shyness, the name is thought to be a derivation of the Greek word *thymon,* meaning "courage." Thyme is the first herb listed in the Holy Herb Charm recited by those with "herb cunning" in the Middle Ages. It has antispasmodic, expectorant, and sedative properties, and its constituent, thymol, a strong antiseptic and germicide, is a major ingredient in Listerine! According to legend, thyme sprouted from the tears of Helen of Troy.

Part used for tea: Leaves
Taste: Pungent, spicy
How to brew: Infuse.
Caution: Excessive use of thyme can lead to symptoms of poisoning and also overstimulate the thyroid. Avoid internal use of the pure essential oil, as it contains thujone (see Caution under Sage, page 139).

health benefits:
* Stimulates production of white blood corpuscles to resist and fight infections
* Relieves flatulence and colic
* Promotes perspiration
* Helpful in throat, bronchial, and lung disorders
* Externally, good as a mouthwash and gargle
* Externally, use to treat fungal infections, such as athlete's foot.

USNEA *(Usnea* spp.)

Known as an herbal antibiotic and antifungal, usnea is really not a plant at all, but a lichen, actually a fungus base, chlorophyll-bearing algae, or two organisms living together in a symbiotic relationship. With such varied historical uses as fodder for caribou, an ingredient in an Icelandic bread recipe, the color for chemists' litmus paper, usnea has also been used for its antibacterial actions to treat urinary and respiratory infections. Known also as "Old Man's Beard," usnea hangs in gray-green strands from pine, oak, fir, and fruit trees in the Northern Hemisphere.

Part used for tea: Whole plant
Taste: Mossy, earthy, slightly astringent
How to brew: Usnic acid, a major medicinal ingredient in usnea, is not very water soluble, so usnea is best added to infusions as a fresh tincture, available in most health food stores.

health benefits:
* Strengthens immune system
* Fights fungal infections such as ringworm and athlete's foot
* Offers support to the body's natural defenses
* Eases symptoms of lupus, an autoimmune disease
* Helps in treating trichomoniasis, a parasitic vaginal infection

health benefits:

* Relieves anxiety, encourages sleep, and improves sleep quality

* Eases muscle spasms, especially shoulder and neck tension

* Reduces mental overactivity and nervous excitability

* Helpful in treating irritable bowel syndrome and stomach and menstrual cramps

* Improves attention span and muscle coordination in children with learning disabilities

Vanilla Orange Honey

This honey is wonderful in herbal teas and can also be used on toast, muffins, scones, and the like! Stir ½ teaspoon vanilla extract and 2 drops pure orange essential oil into ½ cup honey. Stir well. This is unbelievably delicious, makes a great gift, and qualifies as a "love arouser" with definitely exotic aphrodisiac qualities. Try some over vanilla ice cream and then kiss someone you love!

VALERIAN *(Valeriana officinalis)*

Herbalists have, for centuries, recommended this tranquilizing herb for all ailments of the nervous system, such as migraine, hysteria, vertigo, anxiety, insomnia, and convulsions. The name valerian is believed to come from the Latin *valere,* meaning "to be powerful or of well being." The ancient Greek herbalist and physician Dioscorides called it "phu" because of its terrible smell, something like old gym socks!

Part used for tea: Fresh root is best. As it dries, it becomes less sedative and more stimulating.

Taste: Very unusual, aromatic, earthy, distinctive. It is possible to get used to the taste, over time! If using tea or tincture, add some lemon verbena, spearmint, and fresh orange slices to greatly improve the flavor.

How to brew: Decoct or infuse.

Caution: Valerian may cause side effects such as headache and palpitations, and it should not be used during pregnancy. For approximately 25 percent of the population, dried valerian may be stimulating rather than sedative. The fresh herb is more sedative.

VANILLA *(Vanilla planifolia)*

Imported by the Spaniards, vanilla was used for centuries by the Aztec Indians in Mexico. In 1520, it was recorded that ground vanilla was added to the chocolate drink served to the emperor Montezuma, and it has a long history of culinary use in drinks, liqueurs, and desserts. The name, *vaina,* means "pod." Vanilla is one of the most expensive spices in the world due to the lengthy and complicated curing process, selling for as much as $150 to $200 per pound. While there are no known medicinal benefits, it is reputed to have aphrodisiac qualities, enhance the flavor of tea blends, and generally make people happy!

Part used for tea: Pod or extract

Taste: Mellow, fragrant, sweet, delicious

How to brew: Steep chopped pod or add a dash of vanilla extract.

VIOLET (*Viola odorata, V. tricolor,* and spp.)

Traditionally worn by Greeks to keep anger at bay, violet has also been worn as a garland to prevent headaches and dizziness. Ancient Greeks revered it as a symbol of fertility, and Napoleon used it as the emblem of his Imperial party. Both leaves and flowers have antiseptic, diuretic, demulcent, antispasmodic, and expectorant properties, and contain methyl salicylate, an aspirin-like compound. The flowers and leaves contain an abundance of vitamins A and C and are used in Chinese medicine for cleansing lymph and clearing heat in breast cancer treatment. It's the state flower of Illinois, New Jersey, Rhode Island, and Wisconsin. Legend says that drinking violet water inspires love. Distilled water of violets is still available today in apothecaries for use as an enchanting facial toner and cologne.

Part used for tea: Leaves and flowers
Taste: Bland, slightly like wintergreen
How to brew: Infuse.
Caution: Fresh violets can slightly irritate the mucous membranes of the throat with traces of saponins, which break down when the plant is dried or cooked. Eating large quantities of the seeds can cause vomiting.

health benefits:

* Nourishes and builds blood
* Cleanses blood and lymph
* Eases respiratory problems such as bronchitis and cough
* Use as a gargle to soothe throat irritation
* Soothes nerves, headaches, and insomnia
* Has mild laxative action
* Externally, good in facial steams

VITEX (*Vitex agnus-castus*)

Well known in ancient times and featured in Homer's *Iliad,* vitex was imbued with powers to ward off evil. Its common name is chaste tree, and both *agnus* and *castus* mean "chaste." The name is also reputed to have come from the custom of strewing the beds of virgins with vitex leaves during the feast of the harvest goddess. The smell was so bad it was supposed to keep men away! A symbol of chastity, vitex is also thought to reduce sexual desire and unwanted libido in men. It was called "Monk's Pepper" in olden monasteries where it was used as pepper on food, thought to reduce sexual desire. Vitex helps to normalize production of hormones, especially progesterone.

Part used for tea: Berries
Taste: Hot and peppery, similar to black pepper
How to brew: Infuse crushed berries or decoct whole fruit.

health benefits:

* Nourishes and balances the endocrine system, easing symptoms of PMS and menopause
* Regulates menstrual flow
* Aids in balancing hormones and establishing healthy fertility
* Increases breast milk production
* Helps resolve certain types of reproductive cysts and tumors

health benefits:

- Useful in onset of colds and flu
- Relieves symptoms of hay fever
- Eases menstrual cramps and helps reduce heavy menses
- Stimulates weak digestion
- Helps lower high blood pressure, used in formula with other herbs such as hawthorn and motherwort
- Tones varicose veins
- Leaves and flowers, either fresh or dried, can be used as a poultice and hemostat

health benefits:

- Purifies blood, easing skin disorders such as psoriasis, herpes, eczema, and acne
- Stimulates liver and helps regulate bowel movements with mild laxative properties
- Builds red blood cells and raises hematocrit in pregnant women, mixing especially well with nettles and red raspberry
- Eases PMS symptoms

YARROW *(Achillea millefolium)*

The name is derived from Greek mythology, when Achilles put the plant's healing virtues to work on his warriors' battle wounds. Another name for yarrow is *herba militarsa* because it was used so frequently to staunch the wounds of war. The second part of yarrow's name, *millefolium,* means "a thousand leaves," referring to the finely cut foliage. Yarrow has been an important first-aid treatment through the centuries, its very astringency helps to stem the flow of both internal and external bleeding. It provides antispasmodic, anti-inflammatory, and antiallergenic properties as well. Legend says that mixing yarrow with olive oil and applying it to the head prevents baldness.

Part used for tea: Flowers

Taste: Astringent, bitter, earthy

How to brew: Infuse flowers for tea or tincture, and use leaves and flowers for salves and poultices, as the leaves are more bitter than the flowers.

Caution: Large doses of yarrow should not be used during pregnancy, as it is too strong and bitter.

YELLOW DOCK *(Rumex crispus)*

A medicinal plant since ancient times, yellow dock has been valued primarily as a blood purifier, used for chronic skin disorders. So called because of its bright yellow roots, yellow dock is high in iron and also helps the body absorb iron from other food sources, proving useful in treating anemia. This plant is also high in vitamins A and C, and its tannin content is strong enough to tan leather! It has astringent, anti-inflammatory, and tonic properties as well.

Part used for tea: Root (Young leaves are edible raw or cooked.)

Taste: Pleasantly bitter

How to brew: Decoct chopped root.

Caution: Yellow dock leaves contain oxalic acid and prevent absorption of calcium, so use sparingly. The young leaves are fine, a traditional spring green like spinach, chard, beet greens, and the like. Just don't eat it every day.

YERBA BUENA (*Satureja douglasii*)

Yerba buena is a lovely, fragrant member of the mint family. It's found primarily in shady redwood forests from southern California all the way north to British Columbia, but is most commonly found between Santa Barbara and southern Oregon. The original name for San Francisco was *yerba buena,* which means "good herb" in Spanish. Historically, yerba buena was used by Indian tribes and settlers for fevers, colds, and stomach complaints, with both diaphoretic and carminative properties. It is so delicious and refreshing that it has made its way into modern times as a wonderful iced tea. Yerba buena is also used as a flavoring for other less tasty herb blends that need some help going down.

Part used for tea: Leaves
Taste: Delightful, refreshing, like delicate spearmint
How to brew: Infuse (never boil!).
Caution: Be careful that you have the correct plant if picking yerba buena in the wild, and avoid the poison oak growing nearby. If wildcrafting, pick ethically. Be gentle with the plant, and don't rip the roots out of the ground. It's a delicate and special plant.

health benefits:
- Aids digestion and relieves gas and stomachaches
- Promotes sound sleep
- Relieves colds and flu
- Cleanses and stimulates skin, good in facial steams and baths
- Dry and add to herbal potpourris and dream pillows

YERBA SANTA (*Eriodictyon californicum*)

The name of this herb means "holy herb," given by the Spanish after learning of the healing value from Native Americans who chewed or smoked it as a cure for asthma. Tribes in northern California rolled this herb into balls and let them dry in the sun. After chewing the dried balls, they would drink water, creating a natural mouthwash. Many Native American tribes also valued yerba santa as a reliable antiseptic and expectorant for upper respiratory infections. Yerba santa was introduced to the medical profession in 1875, and, after being researched by Parke-Davis, it appeared in *The U.S. Pharmacopoeia* from 1894 to 1905 and again from 1916 to 1947.

Part used for tea: Leaves
Taste: Pleasant, bittersweet, resinous, a bit strawberry-like
How to brew: Infuse or tincture.

health benefits:
- Relieves upper respiratory congestion in coughs, colds, bronchitis, laryngitis, and sore throats
- Helps reduce inflammation and tone mucous membranes during colds, allergy attacks, and sinus infections
- Purifies blood
- Reduces fever

RESOURCES

Seeds & Garden Supplies

Abundant Life Seed Foundation
P.O. Box 772
Port Townsend, WA 98368
(206) 385-5660
Fax (206) 385-7455

Bountiful Gardens
18001 Shafer Ranch Road
Willits, CA 95490

Companion Plants
7297 North Coolville Ridge Road
Athens, OH 45701
(614) 592-4643

Elixir Farm Botanicals LLC
Brixey, MO 65618
(417) 261-2393
Web site http://trine.com/
GardenNet/ElixerFarm/
efb.htm

Gardens Alive! Inc.
5100 Schenley Place
Lawrenceburg, IN 47006
(812) 537-8650
Fax (812) 537-8660

Johnny's Selected Seeds
310 Foss Hill Road
Albion, ME 04910
(207) 437-9294
Fax (207) 437-2165
e-mail janika@johnnyseeds.com

Nichols Garden Nursery
1190 North Pacific Highway
Albany, OR 97321
(503) 967-8406
Fax (503) 928-9280

Renaissance Acres
4450 Valentine
Whitmore Lake, MI 48189
(313) 449-8336
Web site http://www.apin.com/herb

Richter's
Goodwood
Ontario, Canada LOC 1AO
(416) 640-6677
Fax (416) 640-6641

Seeds of Change
1364 Rufina Circle #5
Santa Fe, NM 87501
(505) 983-8956
Fax (505) 983-8957

Herbs & Natural Products

Aspen Hill Farms
1878 Anderson Road, Box 753
Boyne City, MI 49712
(616) 582-6790

Avena Botanicals
219 Mill Street
Rockport, ME 04856
(207) 594-0694

Dry Creek Herb Farm
13935 Dry Creek Road
Auburn, CA 95602
(530) 878-2441
Fax (530) 878-6772

Herb Network
P.O. Box 12937
Albuquerque, NM 87195
Fax (505) 452-8615
e-mail komara@unm.edu

Jean's Greens
R.R. 1, Box 55J
Hale Road
Rensselaerville, NY 12147
(999) 845-8327
Fax (315) 845-6501

Motherlove Herbal Company
P.O. Box 101
LaPorte, CO 80535
(970) 493-2892
Fax (970) 224-4844

Mountain Rose Herbs
P.O. Box 2000
Redway, CA 95560
(800) 879-3337
Fax (707) 923-7867

Pacific Botanicals
4350 Fish Hatchery Road
Grants Pass, OR 97527
Fax (503) 479-5271

Sage Woman Herbs
2211 West Colorado Avenue
Colorado Springs, CO 80904
(719) 473-9702
Fax (719) 473-8873
Web site www.Funtimes.com/
sagewoman.html

San Francisco Herb & Natural Foods Co.
P.O. Box 40604
San Francisco, CA 94140
(510) 547-6345
Fax (510) 547-4234

RESOURCE BOOKS

Avigo, Rosita and Dr. Michael Balick. *Rainforest Remedies: One Hundred Healing Herbs of Belize.* Twin Lakes, WI: Lotus Light Publications, 1993.

Beston, Henry. *Herbs and the Earth.* Boston: David R. Godine, 1995.

Bremness, Lesley. *The Complete Book of Herbs.* New York: Viking Press, 1988.

Bove, Mary. *Herbs for Women's Health: Herbal Help for the Female Cycle from PMS to Menopause.* New Caanan, CT: Keats, 1997.

Bown, Deni. *Encyclopedia of Herbs and Their Uses.* New York: DK Publishing, 1995.

Chevallier, Andrew. *The Encyclopedia of Medicinal Plants.* New York: DK Publishing, 1996.

Crawford, Amanda McQuade. *The Herbal Menopause Book.* Freedom, CA: Crossing Press, 1996.

DeBaggio, Thomas. *Growing Herbs from Seed, Cutting & Root: An Adventure in Small Miracles.* Loveland, CO: Interweave Press, 1995.

De Luca, Diana. *Botanica Erotica: Arousing Body, Mind, and Spirit.* Rochester, VT: Healing Arts Press, 1998.

Duke, James. *The Green Pharmacy.* Emmaus, PA: Rodale Press, 1997.

Foster, Steven. *101 Medicinal Herbs: An Illustrated Guide.* Loveland, CO: Interweave Press, 1998.

Gladstar, Rosemary. *Herbal Healing for Women: Simple Home Remedies for Women of All Ages.* New York: Fireside, 1993.

Green, James. *The Male Herbal Health Care for Men.* Freedom, CA: Crossing Press, 1991.

Grieve, Maud. *A Modern Herbal.* New York: Dover Publications, 1978.

Hill, Madelene and Gwen Barclay. *Southern Herb Growing.* Fredericksberg, TX: Shearer Pub., 1997.

Hobbs, Christopher. *Handbook for Herbal Healing: A Concise Guide to Herbal Products.* New York: Culinary Arts Ltd., 1994.

Hoffman, David. *The New Holistic Herbal.* Rockport, MA: Element, 1991.

Jacobs, Betty E.M. *Growing and Using Herbs Successfully.* Pownal, VT: Storey Books, 1981.

Keville, Kathi. *Herbs for Health and Healing.* Emmaus, PA: Rodale Press, 1996.

Levy, Juliette de Bairacli. *Common Herbs for Natural Health.* Woodstock, NY: Ash Tree Pub., 1997.

Lust, John. *The Herb Book.* New York: Bantam Books, 1983.

Mabey, Richard. *The New Age Herbalist: How to Use Herbs for Healing, Nutrition, Body Care, and Relaxation.* New York: Collier Books, 1988.

Mars, Brigitte. *Herbal Pharmacy* (CD-ROM). Boulder, CO: Hale Software, Inc., 1998.

Murray, Michael. *The Healing Power of Herbs: The Enlightened Person's Guide to the Wonders of Medicinal Plants.* Rocklin, CA: Prima Publishing, 1995.

Ody, Penelope. *The Complete Medicinal Herbal.* New York: DK Publishing, 1993.

Shaudys, Phyllis. *Herbal Treasures: Inspiring Month-By-Month Projects for Gardening, Cooking, and Crafts.* Pownal, VT: Storey Books, 1990.

———. *The Pleasure of Herbs: A Month-By-Month Guide to Growing, Using and Enjoying Herbs.* Pownal, VT: Storey Books, 1986.

Simmons, Adelma G. *Herb Gardening in Five Seasons.* New York: Plume, 1992.

Soule, Deb. *Roots of Healing: A Woman's Book of Herbs.* New York: Citadel Press Books, 1994.

Tyler, Varro. *Herbs of Choice: The Therapeutic Use of Phytomedicinals.* New York: Haworth Press, 1994.

———. *The Honest Herbal: A Sensible Guide to the Use of Herbs and Related Remedies.* New York: Pharmaceutical Press, 1992.

Weed, Susun. *Menopausal Years: The Wise Woman Way, Alternative Approaches for Women 30–90.* Woodstock, NY: Ash Tree Pub., 1992.

INDEX

Page numbers in *italics* indicate photos. Entries in **boldface** indicate recipes.

OTHER STOREY TITLES YOU WILL ENJOY

The Book of Green Tea, by Diana Rosen. A comprehensive guide to the history, varieties, and health benefits of this traditional and enjoyable Asian beverage. Includes recipes for food and beauty and health care products. 160 pages. Paperback. ISBN 1-58017-090-0.

Chai: The Spice Tea of India, by Diana Rosen. Author Diana Rosen uncovers the history of this "common people's drink" while providing recipes for making and cooking with chai and serving suggestions for tea celebrations. Readers will find variations like flavored chai, herbal chai, iced chai, and chai latte and cappuccino, plus recipes for masala cake, cardamom cookies, and chai scones. 160 pages. Paperback. ISBN 1-58017-166-4.

Healing with Herbs, by Penelope Ody. This visual introduction to the world of herbal medicine offers clear, illustrated instructions for growing, preparing, and administering healing herbs to relieve ailments such as arthritis, asthma, ear infections, sinusitis, depression, headaches, infertility, colds, fever, acne, eczema, allergies, and many more. 160 pages. Hardcover. ISBN 1-58017-144-3.

The Herbal Home Remedy Book, by Joyce A. Wardwell. Readers will discover how to use 25 common herbs to make simple herbal remedies. Native American legends and folklore are spread throughout the book. 176 pages. Paperback. ISBN 1-58017-016-1.

Herbal Remedy Gardens, by Dorie Byers. Using simple organic gardening techniques, anyone can grow a healing garden of more than 20 medicinal herbs like garlic, dill, peppermint, and echinacea. Readers will also find recipes, tips for using medicinal herbs, and plans for gardens customized for specific health requirements. 224 pages. Paperback. ISBN 1-58017-095-1.

Herbal Tea Gardens, by Marietta Marshall Marcin. This tea lover's gardening bible contains full instructions for growing and brewing tea herbs plus more than 100 recipes that make use of their healthful qualities. Readers will find complete plans for customized gardens suitable for plots or containers. 192 pages. Paperback. ISBN 1-58017-106-0.

Steeped in Tea, by Diana Rosen. Using a room-by-room approach, this book explores both the drinking and nondrinking uses for tea, including decorating and crafting with tea, making tea health and beauty products and gifts, and creating special places to truly savor the tea-taking experience. Suggestions for traditional tea events and theme tea gardens are also included. 180 pages. Paperback. ISBN 1-58017-093-5.

These books and other Storey Books are available at your bookstore, farm store, garden center,
or directly from Storey Books, Schoolhouse Road, Pownal, Vermont 05261, or by calling 1-800-441-5700.
Or visit our Web site at www.storey.com.